Finding the Best Dentist For Your Child

Treating Children, Not Teeth

Dr. Jack Maltz

ISBN: 978-1-77277-045-2

PUBLISHED BY:
10-10-10 PUBLISHING
MARKHAM, ON
CANADA

Contents

All ideas and thought in this book are my own,
and I have no relationship with any company and
institution that any relationship to this book.

Foreword

Dr. Jack Maltz is a Pediatric Dentist and a teacher. Perhaps this explains his idea for a book that can be read by both layman and dentist, one that begins with how to select the best dentist for the "dental home" that will be your baby's dentist from now until adulthood.

Dr. Maltz goes into great details to release the answers that every mother and father need to help their baby to avoid the scourge of the dental world. Otherwise known as dental caries, tooth decay is a battle hard-fought by the child, even unto adulthood. *Finding The Best Dentist For Your Child* provides tips on how to avoid dental caries, as well as an outline of various treatments available at your dental home. Dr Maltz also describes unusual problems, and how they occur and what the pediatric dentist can do for you.

Having had the pleasure of reading *Finding The Best Dentist For Your Child*, I am convinced of three things. First, all new parents need a copy of this book. Second, if one is available to you, make your children's dentist a pediatric dentist. And third, Dr. Maltz has written a timely and important treatise on dentistry; it should be required reading for those pediatric dentists who are still building their practice.

Raymond Aaron
New York Times Bestselling Author

Introduction

Why Should You Consider Pediatric Dentistry?

The purpose for writing this book is to inform concerned parents about the benefits of choosing a pediatric dentist for your child. First of all, there is a lot of misinformation out there, especially on the internet, about things like: the safety of amalgam (silver) fillings, the question of whether or not to use fluoride, the maximum amount of dental x-rays a child can safely be exposed to, the effects on the teeth from sugar in the diet and even if baby teeth needing fixing. A pediatric dentist can answer such questions and many more—just as I will throughout this book Second, not all doctors/dentists are equal, and everybody has strengths and weaknesses. So, I will answer the questions of how to, why you should and where you can find a good dentist for your kids.

Third, you may not realize it, but there are countless, true horror stories of children being mishandled by dentists. Some have even died. It may not be the case for you, but I'm not at all surprised that dentists are typically feared by parents. Consider these four stories ...

* * *

1. A Florida dentist has been accused of harming the most vulnerable of patients—young children. While doing so, he apparently collected millions of dollars in Medicaid payments for procedures that his patients didn't need or want.

Going to the dentist can be a terrifying experience for children, but some parents say they were horrified when they found out what happened to their kids at the hands of a 78 year-old Jacksonville dentist. In fact, parents are so upset there have been protests outside his practice. One patient was so angry that she was seen attacking him outside his office.

The firestorm started after a mother wrote about the day she took her six year-old daughter to the dentist to have one tooth pulled. On the day of surgery her mother says she was told that she could not sit in the operating room with her daughter.

The woman said she sat in the dentist's office for three hours until the waiting turned to worrying.

"Finally, the nurse came and got me and she said there had been an incident. She was hyperventilating. She had marks all over her, blood all over her."

Angry and unable to get a clear explanation of what happened, the woman says she and her daughter left and rushed to emergency at the nearest hospital.

"In the parking lot, my daughter took her gauze out, and I noticed that all of her teeth were gone."

The mother said the dentist had pulled not one tooth but seven.

Even worse was the report that the doctor had hit her daughter and choked her.

"I decided to put her pictures on Facebook and tell everybody what happened," said the mother. Her story went viral, and other parents started sharing their children's horror stories. A number of civil suits and a criminal case are pending.

"This is somebody who is performing procedures that children don't need, pulling teeth that he knows should be in the child's mouth and who shows patterns of abuse of his child patients," she said.

"My hope is for him to go to jail, to never work on any other kids, and to shut his doors so he can never do this again," said one man.

* * *

2. A 12-year-old Maryland boy, after his dental problems went untreated, succumbed to a severe brain infection. His life could have been spared if his infected tooth was simply removed—a procedure costing just $80. However, the family faced obstacles with Medicaid, poverty and access to resources.

    In the end, once the problem turned deadly, the boy endured two surgeries and weeks of hospital care totaling about $250,000 in medical bills. Sadly, it was too late to save the boy.

    But this boy's story is about more than just a tragic death. His story underscores the growing need in the United States to provide adequate dental care to this nation's children.

Children without Dental Care

Data from the Centers for Disease Control cites tooth decay as one of the most common chronic infectious diseases among U.S. children. By the age of 11, approximately half of America's children have decay, and by the age of 19, tooth decay in the permanent teeth affects about 68 percent of adolescents. For children in low-income families there is nearly twice the risk for untreated tooth decay.

One dental expert says, "Among children, dental services are the most needed service that they do not receive. I think it is probably the least covered of our health benefits across the nation."

Hurdles in Getting Dental Care

While this lack of care is a known problem, there are a number of issues that stand in the way.

First of all, the dentist doesn't break even. In fact, experts say the low rates Medicaid offers to cover dental services are less than what it costs the doctor to do the actual treatment.

Additionally, state Medicaid programs provide less than satisfactory resources for patients seeking dental care. It often happens that when you have the benefits you can't find a dentist to give you care. Then, when a dentist can be found, typically they can't provide the resources required.

The problem with care extends further than bureaucracy, however. I think that, for the general public, dental care is lower down on their list of important issues.

Case for Prevention

People seem to think teeth are not a big deal. But it's not just about your mouth. Infections in your teeth and mouth can lead to more problems. When a cavity goes untreated for months or years, the decay eats the center of the tooth and eventually enters the nerves and blood vessels. From there, bacteria get into the blood stream and can travel virtually anywhere.

By taking advantage of basic preventative services—like cleanings and filling cavities—people can drastically reduce their chances for severe dental disease. But it takes education to help.

* * *

3. A Hawaiian toddler who had no underlying heart problems and suffered a heart attack during a dentist visit likely died because of the drugs used to sedate her, authorities said.

    The three year-old girl lapsed into a coma during the dental procedure in the doctor's office. She died a month later.

    The Honolulu Chief Medical Examiner said that the girl received five drugs in preparation of cavity fillings and root canals: Demerol, hydroxyzine, chlorohydrate, laughing gas and a local anesthetic, lidocaine with epinephrine.

    Apparently, the decedent became unresponsive and went into cardiopulmonary arrest immediately following the lidocaine injection.

    The previously healthy girl's parents filed a negligence lawsuit while she was in a coma.

The death has been classified as an accident, and the doctor's attorney said the allegations were unproven. Nevertheless, the doctor's office is now closed permanently.

* * *

4. A British Columbia dental surgeon failed to properly monitor a young patient who went into cardiac arrest and suffered severe brain damage, the province's regulatory authority for dentists has ruled.

    A discipline panel of the College of Dental Surgeons of B.C. said in a written decision that the dentist involved provided deep sedation using three drugs without being approved to perform such a procedure.

    The patient identified only as HZ went to the Kamloops Oral Surgery and Implant Centre in November 2012 to have her wisdom teeth removed, the college said.

    It said that a monitor showed HZ was experiencing significant cardiac trouble but the doctor continued extracting a tooth and that even when he took action, it was inadequate for a patient who had no pulse.

    A certified dental assistant asked if she should start CPR, and the dentist told her to go ahead while instructing another assistant to call 911 and bring in equipment so he could ventilate HZ. But she had trouble finding the ventilator, the decision said.

    When it was located, it did not fit HZ properly and "he did not hook it up to an oxygen source" or administer the drug epinephrine, which was later given to the patient by ambulance attendants, the college said.

"The panel has concluded that the doctor failed to exercise the level of care, skill and knowledge of a competent practitioner in that he failed to recognize Ms. HZ's cardiac arrest in a timely way and delayed resuscitative measures as a result," the ruling said.

The ruling also said the doctor would leave a sedated patient in order to attend to another patient in his busy practice, where he performed five or six surgeries in a morning.

"Even his certified dental assistant cut corners in that she left a patient who was coming out of sedation to wash her instruments, presumably to prepare for the next surgery."

The decision said the dentist was authorized to provide moderate sedation only. An expert witness told the panel that dentist regularly administered a powerful combination of three drugs in rapid succession, without waiting to observe their impact on a patient and making any necessary adjustments for weight and age.

He continues to practice, with sedation limits imposed by the college, pending the outcome of a hearing that will determine a penalty.[1]

* * *

We, as parents, want to know our children are going to be safe when they go to see a dentist. Most dentists are not like the ones just described, but neither are they the best overall choice for your child. Why? Because a regular dentist is like a general physician: he or she may know a lot about dentistry, but they are not trained to deal with the special problems that can arise with children. A pediatric dentist is. He or she is a specialist dedicated to the oral health of children from infancy through the teen years and has the experience and qualifications to care for a child's teeth, gums and mouth throughout the various stages of childhood.

Children begin to get their baby teeth during the first six months of life. By age six or seven years, they start to lose their first set of teeth, which eventually are replaced by secondary, permanent teeth. Without proper dental care, children face possible oral decay and disease that can cause a lifetime of pain and complications. Today, early childhood dental caries—an infectious disease—is five times more common in children than asthma and seven times more common than hay fever. A pediatric dentist is aware of these things and has received special training to deal with them.

* * *

Getting back to the horror stories we began with, basically, as a parent you have three options when it comes to picking a dentist to do work on young or uncooperative children. I am here to show you the right option and how to know you are actually getting the safest and best results.

The three choices parents have when they have young or uncooperative children are:

1) Do nothing. The problem with this solution is that dental caries is a continual deteriorating situation, in which treatment will get more difficult, more painful and more expensive.
2) Try and do the work in the dental office using sedation and/or sedation and restraints, which may not be safe when using sharp instruments on a fighting, struggling child
3) Have the child put to sleep to complete all the work at one sitting, either in a hospital or in a dental office, with adequate

equipment and personnel. The dentist cannot do both the anaesthesia and the dental work, so there must be an anaesthesiologist, a dentist, a dental assistant and a recovery nurse—at a minimum for safety reasons.

This information needs to be distributed. I do not want to scare people regarding putting their kids to sleep, because when it is done in a proper fashion by competent doctors, it is a safe and routine procedure that is carried out hundreds of times per day. But neither should you be unaware of the risks your child faces if the wrong choice is made.

Some basic information regarding pediatric dentists follows.

What Kinds of Training Do Pediatric Dentists Have?

Pediatric dentists have completed at least
- Two-four years of dental school
- Two-three additional years of residency training in dentistry for infants, children, teens, and children with special needs

What Types of Treatments Do Pediatric Dentists Provide?

Pediatric dentists provide comprehensive oral health care that includes the following:
- Infant oral health exams, which include risk assessment for dental caries in mother and child
- Preventive dental care including cleaning and fluoride treatments, as well as nutrition and diet recommendations
- Habit counseling (for example, pacifier use and thumb sucking)
- Early assessment and possible treatment for straightening teeth and correcting an improper bite (orthodontics)

- Repair of tooth cavities or defects
- Diagnosis of oral conditions associated with diseases such as diabetes, congenital heart defect, asthma, hay fever, and attention deficit/ hyperactivity disorder
- Management of gum diseases and conditions, including ulcers, short frenulae, mucoceles and pediatric periodontal disease
- Care for dental injuries (for example, fractured, displaced, or knocked-out teeth)

Where Can I Find a Pediatric Dentist?

Pediatric dentists practice in a variety of locations including private practices, dental schools, and medical centers. Your pediatrician can help you find a pediatric dentist near your home.

In Ontario, a pediatric dentist can be found at the following Ontario Dental Association registry: http://www.youroral health.ca/find-a-dentist24

In Canada, the National Voice of Pediatric Dentistry can be found at http://www.capd-acdp.org/

In the United States, the American Academy of Pediatric Dentistry offers a similar service at: http://www.aapd.org/

(More on this later.)

Pediatric Dentists—the Best Care for Children

Children are not just small adults. They are not always able to be patient and cooperative during a dental exam. Pediatric dentists know how to examine and treat children in ways that make them comfortable. In addition, pediatric dentists use specially designed equipment in offices that are arranged and decorated with children in mind.

A pediatric dentist offers a wide range of treatment options, as well as expertise and training to care for your child's teeth, gums, and mouth. When your pediatrician suggests that your child receive a dental exam, you can be assured that a pediatric dentist will provide the best possible care.

[1] http://www.ctvnews.ca/health/b-c-dentist-caused-patient-to-suffer-brain-damage-panel-1.2460230

Chapter One
The Importance of Primary Teeth

Caring for Baby Teeth

It's the middle of the night and your child is wailing. Nothing you do can get her settled. The problem is likely teeth. You can't see them. But they're there. Baby teeth ... they started forming way back in the womb, but before you know it they'll be erupting through your baby's gums. What she needs is for you to gently rub her gums with a clean finger, a wet gauze pad or a small, cool spoon. You can also offer a cold washcloth to chew on or a rubber teething ring, something to chew on to dull the pain. You might even need to give your baby some Tylenol or Advil.

* * *

The first baby teeth, known as primary teeth, start to erupt through the gums between the ages of six months to one year of age. The timing will vary, but all 20 primary teeth will usually erupt by the age of three. And those baby teeth are important, even if you can't see them and even if they eventually fall out and are replaced with permanent adult teeth. Baby teeth are in fact, extremely important.

The Importance of Primary Teeth

- For appearance, esthetics
- Chewing, eating, mastication, swallowing
- General good health, speech
- Jaw and facial development
- Hold spot for permanent teeth

And baby teeth are just as prone to cavities as adult teeth. In fact, more than 50 percent of children will be affected by tooth decay before age five. So, you want to keep those cavities away to avoid an early loss of a tooth. When a baby tooth is lost too early, the permanent teeth can drift into the empty space and make it difficult for other adult teeth to find room when it's their turn to erupt. So, proper oral hygiene is important as soon as your baby is born. Establishing good oral habits early will go a long way, even beyond impressing the tooth fairy!

Teething

When baby teeth emerge through the gum, it's called teething. It can be a bit painful, and it can make your child cranky. But, it's a very natural process that every developing child goes through. Your baby's gums may be sore and tender, and they may drool a bit. But, as previously mentioned, there are ways to alleviate some of that pain and make your baby, and you, feel a whole lot better.

How to Clean Baby Teeth

Good oral hygiene begins at birth. So it's wise to get in the habit of cleaning your baby's gums even before any primary teeth come in. Gently clean your baby's gums after every feeding using a clean, damp washcloth or a toothbrush with soft bristles and a small head made just for babies.

As soon as the first baby tooth arrives, you can start brushing it with a toothbrush and toothpaste. To brush baby teeth, use a small amount of non-fluoride toothpaste (sometimes called training toothpaste). Brush the front and back of your baby's teeth, and lift your baby's lips to make sure you get the gum line. You should brush your baby's teeth twice a day.

Try to have your baby realize that you brush your teeth too. It can greatly influence their desire to brush like you do.

When Should a Baby First See a Dentist?

Your doctor wants you to have a lifetime of smiles. And he wants to be with you throughout that lifetime. That's why he would like you to make his office your dental home. By definition, a dental home is the ongoing relationship between the dentist and the patient; a relationship that begins with the child's very first visit around the age of one and includes all aspects of oral health care delivered in a comprehensive, continuously accessible, coordinated, and family-centered way. It also means you'll be in the hands of a dental specialist if need be. You get that with a Pediatric Dentist, and more. Good habits start early. So, establish your dental home and schedule your child's first dental visit shortly after the first tooth appears and no later than your child's first birthday.

Thumb sucking and Baby Teeth

Thumb sucking is a natural reflex for children. Sucking on thumbs, fingers, pacifiers or anything they can get their mouths on can help babies learn to feel safe and secure. Thumb sucking is a soothing action for babies, and can even help them lull themselves to sleep.

Thumb sucking is all well and good—until your child's permanent teeth come in. Then it can cause problems. Crooked teeth and bite problems can result from thumb sucking. Also, the roof of the mouth can become unnaturally constricted or elevated and the jaws may not develop properly. The intensity of sucking matters, too. Aggressive suckers may even develop problems with their baby teeth.

Children usually stop sucking their thumbs between the ages of two and four years old, or by the time the permanent front teeth are ready to erupt. This is good news for those emerging adult teeth! But if you have trouble getting your child to stop thumb sucking, try the following tips …

How to Stop Thumb sucking

- Limit the time your child sucks their thumb to when they are in their bedroom or only during naptime
- Praise your child for not sucking
- If your child sucks their thumb for comfort, try to correct the cause of anxiety
- Recruit your dentist in encouraging your child to stop thumb sucking
- Remind your child of their thumb sucking habit by putting a sock over their hand when they nap or sleep

Children Oral Hygiene and Diet

Just as it is for adults, good oral hygiene and a well-balanced diet are good for children. It's good for their teeth and it's good for their overall well-being. And good habits start young. So gently clean your baby's gums after every feeding and give your baby healthy foods.

Even though it may be tempting to let your child fall asleep with a baby bottle in their mouth, don't. Letting a baby fall asleep with a bottle full of milk, formula, juice or any sweet drink is like soaking those developing teeth in sugar. That wouldn't be good for anyone's teeth, especially your baby's, and it can result in baby bottle tooth decay. Good oral health and diet is pivotal to establishing a lifetime full of happy, healthy smiles. All it takes is brushing, flossing, and eating right. The key is to start those positive habits at an early age.[2]

Development of Teeth

All twenty baby (or primary) teeth come in by the time your child is two or three years old.

This chart tells you when baby teeth come in (or erupt) in most children.

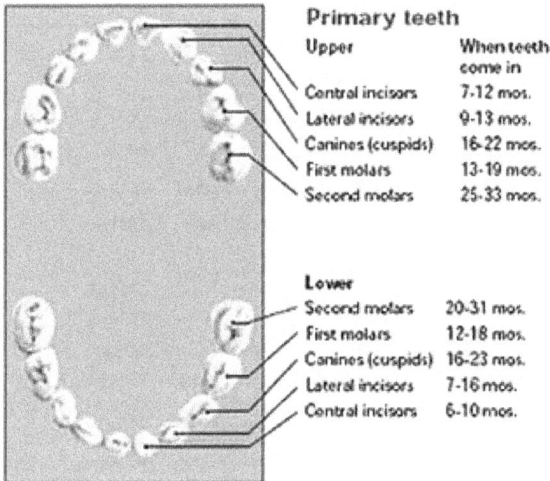

Primary teeth

Upper	When teeth come in
Central incisors	7-12 mos.
Lateral incisors	9-13 mos.
Canines (cuspids)	16-22 mos.
First molars	13-19 mos.
Second molars	25-33 mos.

Lower	
Second molars	20-31 mos.
First molars	12-18 mos.
Canines (cuspids)	16-23 mos.
Lateral incisors	7-16 mos.
Central incisors	6-10 mos.

If your child is getting his or her teeth and seems to be in pain, you can:
- rub the gums with a clean finger, or
- rub the gums with the back of a small, cool spoon.

If your child is still unhappy, your dentist, pharmacist or doctor can suggest an over-the-counter medicine to ease the pain.

Here's what you should not do:
- Do not use the kind of painkiller that can be rubbed on your child's gums. Your child may swallow it.
- Do not give your child teething biscuits. They may have sugar added or contain hidden sugars.

Permanent Teeth

At age six or seven, the first adult (or permanent) teeth come in. They are known as the "first molars," or the "six-year molars." They come in at the back of the mouth, behind the last baby (or primary) teeth. They do not replace any primary teeth.

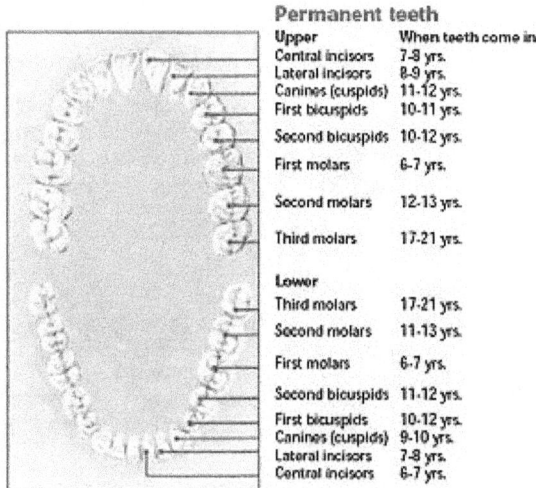

Permanent teeth

Upper	When teeth come in
Central incisors	7-8 yrs.
Lateral incisors	8-9 yrs.
Canines (cuspids)	11-12 yrs.
First bicuspids	10-11 yrs.
Second bicuspids	10-12 yrs.
First molars	6-7 yrs.
Second molars	12-13 yrs.
Third molars	17-21 yrs.

Lower	
Third molars	17-21 yrs.
Second molars	11-13 yrs.
First molars	6-7 yrs.
Second bicuspids	11-12 yrs.
First bicuspids	10-12 yrs.
Canines (cuspids)	9-10 yrs.
Lateral incisors	7-8 yrs.
Central incisors	6-7 yrs.

It's okay for children to wiggle their primary teeth if they are loose. But it's not okay to use force to pull out a tooth that's not ready to come out. When a tooth comes out at the right time, there will be very little bleeding.

Why Do the New Permanent Teeth Look Yellow?

Permanent teeth often look more yellow than primary teeth. This is normal as baby teeth are naturally whiter. But it could also be caused by medicine your child took, by an accident that hurt a primary tooth, or by too much fluoride. Ask your dentist about this when you go for a dental exam.

Healthy Gums

Cavities are the main problem children have with their teeth. But children can get gum disease too, just like adults. It happens when the gums that hold our teeth in place get inflamed.

Daily brushing and flossing can stop gum disease. If your child's gums bleed, don't stop brushing. If the gums are always swollen, sore or bleeding, there may be a serious problem. You should take your child to the dentist. A sign of inflamed gums is bleeding on brushing.

Dental Safety

Here are some ways to protect your child's teeth:

- Always use infant car seats and seat belts when you drive.
- Babies will chew on almost anything. Keep them away from hard things that could crack their teeth.
- Children fall a lot when they are learning to walk. Teeth can break, crack, get knocked out or become loose. See your dentist if this happens.

If you have questions about your child's teeth, talk to your dentist.

What is Tooth Decay (Caries or Cavities)?

Tooth decay (destruction of tooth structure) is the disease known as caries or cavities. Tooth decay is a highly preventable disease caused by bacteria and other factors. It can occur when foods containing carbohydrates (sugars and starches), such as milk, soda, raisins, candy, cake, fruit juices, cereals, and bread, are left on the teeth. Bacteria that normally live in the mouth change these foods, producing acids. The combination of bacteria, food, acid, and saliva form a substance called plaque that sticks to the teeth. Over time, the acids produced by the bacteria eat away at the tooth enamel, causing cavities.

Who is at Risk for Tooth Decay?

We all host bacteria in our mouths which makes everyone a potential target for cavities. Risk factors that put a person at a higher risk for tooth decay include:

- High levels of the bacteria that cause cavities
- Diets high in sweets, carbohydrates, and sugars
- Water supplies with limited or no fluoridation
- Poor oral hygiene
- Reduced salivary flow

What are the Symptoms of Tooth Decay and Dental Caries?

The following are the most common signs and symptoms of tooth decay and dental caries, however, each child may experience them differently. Signs may include white spots on the teeth that appear first. Then, an early cavity appears that has a light brown color on the tooth. The tooth color progressively becomes darker and a hole (cavitation) may appear. Symptoms, such as sensitivity to sweets, cold beverages or foods may occur and eventually pain, but not always.

How is Tooth Decay Diagnosed?

Dental caries is usually diagnosed based on a complete history and physical exam of your child. This may be done by your child's health care provider or your child's dentist—by visual and tactile examination

How Can Tooth Decay Be Prevented?

Preventing tooth decay and cavities involves these simple steps:

- Start brushing your child's teeth as soon as the first one appears. Brush the teeth, tongue, and gums twice a day with a fluoridated toothpaste, or supervise them brushing their teeth.
- For children less than three years-old, use only a small amount of toothpaste.
- Starting at three years of age, use a pea-sized amount of toothpaste.
- Make sure your child eats a well-balanced diet and limit or eliminate sugary snacks.
- Also ask about dental sealants and fluoride varnish. Both are applied to the teeth.
- Schedule routine (every six months) dental cleanings and exams for your child.

What is the Treatment for Tooth Decay?

Treatment, in most cases, requires: a) removing the decayed part of the tooth and replacing it with a filling or b) extracting the tooth.

What are Fillings?

Fillings (also called restorations) are materials placed in teeth to repair damage caused by tooth decay. Advances in dental materials and techniques provide new, effective ways to restore teeth.

A single visit is all that is required to place a filling directly into a prepared cavity or hole. Materials used for these filings include dental amalgam, also known as silver fillings; glass ionomers; resin ionomers; and some composite (resin) fillings.

Amalgam fillings have been used for decades and have been tested for safety and resistance to wear. Dentists have found amalgams to be safe, reliable, and effective for restorations.

Glass ionomers are tooth-colored materials made from fine glass powders and acrylic acids. These are used in small fillings that don't have to withstand heavy pressure from chewing. Resin ionomers are made from glass with acrylic acids and acrylic resin. [3]

Why Treat Baby Teeth?

There are several reasons to fix baby teeth;

1. Every child's smile affects their sense of self-esteem and confidence in life.

2. Primary teeth are important because they help guide proper eruption of the permanent teeth.
3. Primary teeth help maintain good nutrition with proper chewing.
4. Primary teeth help with the development of speech.
5. Untreated baby teeth can affect the development of the permanent teeth.
6. Not treating the teeth can result in a patient with severe pain and possibly developing an abscess.

An abscess "is a collection of pus that has accumulated in a cavity formed within a tissue because of an inflammatory process in response to an infection process, usually caused by bacteria." (Wikipedia)

An abscess can be very dangerous and can lead to swelling and severe pain.

It's Just a Baby Tooth, Pull it!

Many times we encounter the dilemma of "What do we do with baby teeth that have severe decay?" Parents are often surprised when they learn that their child has dental decay. "They are baby teeth. Can't you just pull them?" they say, questioning the need to restore primary teeth.

Let's start by saying that primary teeth or baby teeth serve a very important purpose; they save space for the permanent teeth. The twenty primary teeth are replaced by twenty permanent teeth. If a baby tooth is lost before the permanent tooth is ready to erupt, adjacent teeth will drift and tip into the empty space. This will cause serious space problems when the permanent tooth is ready to come into the space that has been lost.

The primary teeth must be present to help guide the proper path for eruption of the permanent teeth. The anterior teeth are lost naturally between 5-6 years of age. The eight baby molars aren't ready to come out until 9-13 years of age. If a primary second molar is lost too early because decay, the permanent molar that erupts at six years of age will have no guide to its proper position. It will drift forward taking the space of the adjacent un-erupted permanent tooth, blocking it out.

\If a baby tooth has decay your dentist will recommend fillings to prevent spreading of the decay. If the decay is too advanced and the tooth cannot be restored with a filling, the doctor may recommend a stainless steel crown or silver cap. The stainless steel crown provides the tooth with full coverage that is long lasting, until the permanent tooth is ready to erupt.

When the decay travels to the center of the tooth where the nerve and blood vessel lie, a pulpotomy can be performed to remove the decay and infected nerve. If the infection spreads to the bone and causes an abscess, the tooth will need to be extracted. Soon after the extraction a space maintainer should be fabricated to fit the space. The space maintainer is an appliance that is custom fit to the patient's mouth and stays in the child's mouth until the permanent tooth starts to erupt. The appliance will prevent the adjacent teeth from drifting or tipping into the space.

Don't forget to brush to keep that beautiful little smile shining![4]

When Should They Treat Tooth Decay?

What is tooth decay?

Tooth decay refers to the loss of minerals from the tooth structure caused by bacteria.

Why does a tooth become decayed?

When tooth surfaces are covered with dental plaque, the bacteria in the plaque will metabolize the sugars in your food and produce acids which will demineralize the tooth surface.

Saliva can reduce acid attacks towards teeth by neutralizing it and preventing further loss of minerals. However, there must be enough time for saliva to work.

If we eat and drink frequently, saliva will not have enough time to work. The minerals on the tooth surface will continue to lose out, and then tooth decay may occur.

Symptoms and Treatment Methods of Tooth Decay

Early stage of tooth decay
Decay usually occurs at the enamel of the tooth. Early stages of tooth decay are usually painless and the tooth will seem undamaged to the naked eye. Therefore, it is difficult to notice the decay.

Treatment:
The early tooth decay can be prevented by application of concentrated fluoride by a dentist.

Tooth decay spreads into dentine
When tooth decay spreads into dentine, a cavity may appear, and pain is felt when eating.

Treatment:
- A dental filling can be placed when the cavity is small and the bulk of the tooth remains sound.
- A crown can be placed when the cavity is widespread and the remaining tooth is weak.

Tooth decay spreads into the pulp

At this stage, the carious cavity is obvious and causes severe pain. The pulp tissues are infected by the bacteria and may become inflamed or even necrotic. The bacteria may spread from the pulp to the tooth to surrounding tissues via the apex of the tooth, leading to the formation of an abscess.

Treatment:
- Pulp treatment followed by filling, or crown, depending on the condition of the remaining
tooth structure.
- If pulp treatment is not appropriate, an extraction will be necessary.

Consequence of tooth decay
- The decayed cavity emits unpleasant odour and causes bad breath. This directly affects normal social life.
- Tooth decay may lead to persistent pain, which may not be controlled by painkiller and, therefore, affects one's appetite, studies, work and sleep.
- When there is severe tooth decay, the bacteria may spread from the pulp to the tooth to surrounding tissues via the apex of the tooth, leading to the formation of an abscess.
- If a tooth is severely damaged and even pulp treatment is not applicable, an extraction is then necessary. After extraction, the neighbouring teeth may shift towards the empty space and cause malocclusion.

Methods to Prevent Tooth Decay

Keep good dietary habits

Every time we eat, demineralization occurs at the surface of our teeth and creates a chance for getting tooth decay. The more often we eat the more chances we have to get tooth decay.

Therefore, having regular meals three times a day with sufficient amount of food during each meal will reduce the frequency of meals. In addition, drink plain water to quench thirst. This can reduce the chance of getting tooth decay. If you feel hungry in between meals, you may snack once.

Brush your teeth with fluoride toothpaste
Fluoride strengthens the teeth by increasing their resistance to acid attack. Fluoride also facilitates minerals to re-enter the teeth (re-mineralization) and helps restore early tooth decay. Therefore, you should brush in the morning and before bed at night with fluoride toothpaste.

Regular dental check-up
Have a regular dental check-up at least once a year so that tooth decay can be diagnosed at an early stage. Preventive dental treatments such as fissure sealants can be applied.[5]

Oral Development

Tooth eruption may be delayed, accelerated, or inconsistent in children with growth disturbances. Gums may appear red or bluish-purple before erupting teeth break through into the mouth. Eruption depends on genetics, growth of the jaw, muscular action, and other factors. Children with Down syndrome may show delays of up to two years. **Refer to an oral health care provider for additional questions.**

Developmental defects appear as pits, lines, or discoloration in the teeth. Very high fever or certain medications can disturb tooth formation and defects may result. Many teeth with defects are prone to dental caries, are difficult to keep clean, and may compromise appearance. **Refer to an oral health care provider for evaluation of treatment options and advice on keeping teeth clean.**

Tooth anomalies are variations in the number, size, and shape of teeth. People with Down syndrome, oral clefts, ectodermal dysplasias, or other conditions may experience congenitally missing, extra, or malformed teeth. **Consult an oral health care provider for dental treatment planning during a child's growing years.**

Oral Trauma

Trauma to the face and mouth occur more frequently in people who have intellectual disability, seizures, abnormal protective reflexes, or muscle incoordination. People receiving restorative dental care should be observed closely to prevent chewing on anesthetized areas. **If a tooth is avulsed or broken, take the patient and the tooth to a dentist immediately. Counsel the parent/caregiver on ways to prevent trauma and what to do when it occurs.**

Bruxism

Bruxism, the habitual grinding of teeth, is a common occurrence in people with cerebral palsy or severe intellectual disability. In extreme cases, bruxism leads to tooth abrasion and flat biting surfaces.

Oral Infections

Dental caries, or tooth decay, may be linked to less than normal amounts of saliva, medications containing sugar, or special diets that require prolonged bottle feeding or snacking. When oral hygiene is poor, the teeth are at increased risk for caries. **Counsel the parent/caregiver on daily oral hygiene and use of a fluoride-containing toothpaste. Refer to an oral health care provider and/or gastroenterologist for prevention and treatment. Prescribe sugarless medications when available.**

Viral infections are usually due to the herpes simplex virus. Children rarely get herpetic gingivostomatitis or herpes labialis before six months of age. Herpetic gingivostomatitis is most common in young children, but may occur in adolescents and young adults. Viral infections can be painful and are usually accompanied by a fever. **Counsel the parent/caregiver about the infectious nature of the lesions, the need for frequent fluids to prevent dehydration, and methods of symptomatic treatment.**

Tips for Health Care Providers

- Take time to talk and listen to parents and caregivers.
- Tell parents and caregivers to seek a dental consultation no later than a child's first birthday.
- Seek advice on behavior management techniques; early intervention and familiarization with the dental team may take several visits.
- Evaluate and treat orthodontic problems early to minimize risk of more complicated problems later in life.
- Advise caregivers to avoid serving snacks at bedtime.[6]

[2] http://www.dentalassociates.com/pediatric-dentistry/importance-baby-teeth/

[3] http://www.hopkinsmedicine.org/healthlibrary/conditions/pediatrics/tooth_decay_caries_or_cavities_in_children_90,P01848/

[4] http://www.childrensdentalhealth.com/about-you/why-baby-teeth/

[5] http://www.toothclub.gov.hk/en/pnc/en_pnc_2_1_5_1.html
Children with Special Needs and Medical Conditions

[6] http://www.nidcr.nih.gov/oralhealth/OralHealthInformation/ChildrensOralHealth/OralConditionsChildrenSpecialNeeds.htm

Chapter 2
How and why Dental Caries Starts

Dental Caries (Tooth Decay)

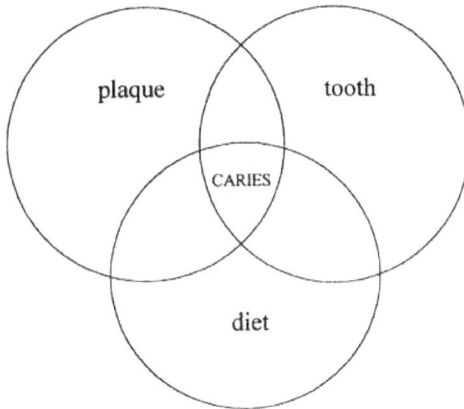

What It Takes to Start Dental Caries (DC)

Note how the above diagram shows the interaction of teeth, germs and sugars. All three are needed to create DC. Some teeth are more prone to DC than others, depending on their position in the mouth. The further back the teeth are, the less likely they are to be well cleaned and deep groves in molars and premolars are predisposed to DC. Also, severe crowding prevents adequate cleaning. It is also true that food and debris accumulation, along with enamel defects, can make teeth more cavity prone, just as newly erupted teeth need special attention.

How and Why Dental Caries Starts

DC is the most common chronic disease of childhood, with 60% of children having significant tooth decay by age 5. The prevalence increases by 17 years of age as 78% of U.S. kids have DC. 90% of DC in school age children occurs in pits and fissures of back teeth (AAPD manual pg 18).

Why Some Kids Get Dental Caries and Some Do Not

Parents often assume that kids get cavities because they're lax about brushing and flossing. That's true to an extent, but what few people know is that tooth decay is a disease known as dental caries which is caused by specific germs, that spread easily within families and that can last a lifetime. What's more, it's more common among young children than any other chronic illness, including asthma and diabetes.

At least 4 million preschoolers suffer from tooth decay—an increase of more than 600,000 kids in the last decade. "Children now have much more sugar in their diets at an early age," says Paul Casamassimo, D.D.S., professor of pediatric dentistry at the Ohio State University College of Medicine and Public Health, in Columbus. The popularity of bottled water—which usually doesn't contain fluoride—may also contribute to the growing problem, he says.

Tooth decay begins with a group of germs called *mutans streptococcus*. "The bacteria feed on sugar and produce acid that eats away at the structure of teeth by depleting calcium," explains Parents advisor Burton Edelstein, D.D.S., founding director of the Children's Dental Health Project. The bacteria also create plaque—a yellowish film that builds up on teeth and contains even more enamel-eroding acid. Once an area without calcium becomes big enough, the surface of the tooth collapses, and that's a cavity.

Babies are born without any of these harmful bacteria in their mouth, and studies have proven that moms (rather than dads) typically infect their children before age two. It happens when you transfer your saliva into your child's mouth—by repeatedly eating from the same spoon as your baby, for example, or letting your toddler brush his teeth with your toothbrush. And if you've frequently had cavities yourself, you're particularly likely to pass the germs along. Once a child's mouth has become colonized with mutans, he'll be prone to cavities in his baby and permanent teeth that can cause pain and difficulty eating. "It's an old wives' tale that 'soft teeth' run in families, but what's really passed along in families are high levels of decay-causing bacteria," says Dr. Edelstein. In fact, 80 percent of all cavities occur in just 25 percent of kids. The key role that bacteria plays in decay may also explain why some kids who eat tons of candy or never floss are lucky enough to avoid dental problems.

Emilie Mosby, of Kingman, Arizona, had lots of cavities when she was a kid, so she panicked when she saw a dark spot on her three year-old daughter's tooth. "I took Teagan to the dentist, and when he told me she had a cavity, I almost cried," says Mosby. "It's so frustrating. I've always tried to take good care of her teeth, and I have a friend who doesn't even brush her kids' teeth every day and they've never gotten cavities."

If you've had trouble with your teeth, you need to take responsibility for your child's dental health—just like you'd be vigilant if you've had a family history of high cholesterol or skin cancer. Unfortunately, antibiotics can't get rid of the cavity-causing bacteria in your child's mouth. That's why the American Academy of Pediatrics (AAP) actually urges pediatricians to ask parents about their own dental history by the time their baby is six months old, and to recommend taking extra precautions if a child is at high risk.[7]

Why Different Dentists Come Up With Different Treatment Plans

No matter how long we have been practicing, we are all guilty of not seeing the forest for the trees.

We all treatment-plan differently, from the perspective of our biases and experiences. This is why the question, *If this was your son/daughter/mother/father/etc., what would you do?* poses such a problem for us all. Emotion clouds judgment, but our diagnostic and problem-solving skills are much better from an objective perspective than a subjective one.

From the moment we walk into our new patient exams, we start formulating these treatment plans based on the problems that are presented. Even while patients describe their problems, most of us are trying to think of ways to solve them right then and there ... not really listening.

We need to listen to our patients and realize that they are telling us what they want and why they are in our chair. This changes because of the type of dentist or dental specialist we might be, but overall, the experience is the same. Where you go from here can define success or problems in each and every case.

I believe that treatment planning is the core of what makes you a good doctor. And here's the real secret: *There is no secret!* Being able to comprehensively treatment-plan a case is the most important principle in dentistry.

What does a **comprehensive treatment plan** mean? What questions do you have to ask? What information do you need to be able to assess and process a treatment plan?

My first question is this. When you are remodeling a house, would you start without an architect or an interior designer? How would you know where the best place is to position everything? Where do the walls go? Where can you place the windows or the floors? ...

I believe that in order to start the process of treatment planning, you need information. You need to assess the patient from a global position. We all have GPS in our cars, and now on our phones. When using your GPS, you need to know your starting position and the destination. During single-tooth dentistry, we all can predict the dentistry that is involved, whether we are prepping a crown, or even the simplest of restorations—an occlusal composite. However, when we are planning someone's smile, we need a destination. All of these processes allow the dentist to plan the smile, or the remodeled house from our analogy above.

You need to start from the outside and work inside. The typical routine for the dentist is to take dental records, which allows this perspective. This is why I believe that the dentist's role in treatment planning is akin to the architect from our construction analogy. The dental records will define the patient's structural limitations (the position of the existing structure/walls). And I always advocate that in your most complex cases, working with a specialist or team of specialists will afford both the dentist (general practitioner) and the patient the best treatment possible. Unfortunately, we are all guilty of looking at the trees without seeing the forest. Believing that dentistry is a team sport and that we are all working toward the same goal will make your dentistry more rewarding and special.

How Does the Dentist Know When to Treat Dental Caries?

Teeth are in an environment of constant acid attack that strips the teeth of important minerals and breaks the teeth down. While this attack is constantly occurring, minerals are also being constantly replenished through mineral-rich saliva and fluoridated water and toothpaste. In addition to fluoride, calcium and phosphate also help to remineralize enamel. When the demineralization starts and is confined to the outermost layer of enamel, it is called an incipient cavity. These types of lesions rarely need anything more than very conservative treatment. Only when the cavity breaks through the enamel layer and into the dentin does it really threaten the tooth. So when these lesions are detected, it is best to try a remineralization protocol to see if they can be reversed instead of jumping to a filling right away. A dentist will help in determining the most effective conservative treatment for these early cavities.

The dentist's goal is to achieve a healthy balance between prevention and restoration. It is a balance between being proactive and reactive. The dentist doesn't want to be so proactive that he is recommending things that don't need to be done—preventing problems that realistically never would have occurred. But he doesn't want to be so reactive that he simply watches small problems become big problems. One mistake people often make is waiting for pain to dictate the timing of treatment. Once a tooth starts hurting, it is often too late for remineralization or a small filling. Pain usually indicates a need for root canal treatment, a crown, or tooth extraction. There is some variability in how dentists will treat microcavities and when they determine a filling is necessary. Some people are more prone to caries than others. Analyzing one's history of cavities, current diet, and oral hygiene may lead the dentist to be more aggressive or more conservative with his recommendations.

Regardless of the dentist, regular returns to the dentist are key to being conservative so the cavity can be monitored and treated before it grows too much. Small cavities can become root canals within a year under the right circumstances. As a cavity grows, more tooth structure is lost. And lost tooth structure leads to a greater likelihood of fractured teeth, recurrent decay, and tooth loss. When possible, one is always better off getting a small filling than ending up with a large filling, a root canal, or a crown.[8]

Baby Teeth Fall Out. Why Do I Need to Fix Them?

Once your child has teeth, he is susceptible to tooth decay. So, lift his or her lips once a month and check the teeth. Look for dull white spots or lines on the teeth. These may be on the necks of the teeth next to the gums. Dark teeth are also a sign of tooth decay.

If you see any signs, go to the dentist right away. Early childhood tooth decay must be treated quickly. If not, your child may have pain and infection.

Do I Really Need a Root Canal for My Child's Baby Teeth?

You might be wondering why your child needs a root canal if one or more of their baby teeth are in danger. Won't their adult teeth just grow in anyways? Children typically shed their baby teeth for adult teeth around 6-12 years old, but this is a big age spread. If your child's tooth is infected and has to be removed and they are only four, it could be seven years before their adult tooth sprouts, leaving them with a gap in their mouth for a long time. In some cases your child's root pulp may be exposed, and this can be very painful. By treating this with a root canal you can provide your child with a solution to the pain and discomfort, while restoring their tooth to its natural appearance. Missing teeth can lead to other problems such as:

- Impacted speech
- Inability to properly chew
- Insecurities about appearance
- Depending on where the missing tooth is located it can be more difficult to brush and floss.
- Missing teeth leave your gums and jawbone exposed to added pressure that can cause damage.

For these reasons, many parents decide that a root canal is the best option for their child. Baby teeth are an important component to your child's developing mouth. Dental professionals highly recommend taking the necessary measures to save baby teeth using root canals whenever possible. After the procedure is complete and a cap is secured on top, this tooth should remain strong and stoic in your child's mouth until the time comes and they lose their tooth. Since the materials used to create a root canal are biocompatible, meaning they work with your body, as soon as the tooth is ready to come loose it will.

Baby Teeth, Caries and Permanent Teeth

There are a number of adult teeth sitting under the baby teeth. Decay and infection does not just stop at the baby teeth. Also, most people misunderstand the importance of a baby tooth. Even though it will eventually be lost, it should be taken care of until it is gone. Sometimes there is no adult tooth to replace the baby tooth—imagine that! So, it is important to develop good habits regarding the care of teeth long before the adult teeth appear.

Parents and Dental Caries

There are studies that show parents are nowhere near reactive enough to the onset of DC in children. Also, DC is a worldwide plague of massive proportions. The only way this can become better is if parents learn to take responsibility for both their dental health and that of their children. It's that simple.

Dental Caries and General Health

Oral health is essential to general health and well-being at every stage of life. A healthy mouth enables not only nutrition of the physical body, but also enhances social interaction and promotes self-esteem and feelings of well-being. The mouth serves as a "window" to the rest of the body, providing signals of general health disorders. For example, mouth lesions may be the first signs of HIV infection, aphthous ulcers are occasionally a manifestation of Coeliac disease or Crohn's disease, pale and bleeding gums can be a marker for blood disorders, bone loss in the lower jaw can be an early indicator of skeletal osteoporosis, and changes in tooth appearance can indicate bulimia or anorexia. The presence of many compounds (e.g., alcohol, nicotine, opiates, drugs, hormones, environmental toxins, antibodies) in the body can also be detected in the saliva. Oral conditions have an impact on overall health and disease. Bacteria from the mouth can cause infection in other parts of the body when the immune system has been compromised by disease or medical treatments (e.g., infective endocarditis). Systemic conditions and their treatment are also known to impact on oral health (e.g., reduced saliva flow, altered balance of oral microorganisms).

Periodontal disease has been associated with a number of systemic conditions. Though the biological interactions between oral conditions such as periodontal disease and other medical conditions are still not fully understood, it is clear that major chronic diseases—namely cancer and heart disease—share common risk factors with oral disease. Recognition that oral health and general health are interlinked is essential for determining appropriate oral health care programmes and strategies at both individual and community care levels. That the mouth and body are integral to each other underscores the importance of the integration of oral health into holistic general health policies and of the adoption of a collaborative "Common Risk Factor Approach" for oral health promotion.

The Common Risk Factor Approach

Traditionally, oral health promotion has focused on the care of the teeth and gums, in isolation from other health programmes. The Common Risk Factor Approach (CRFA) to health promotion takes a broader perspective and targets risk factors common to many chronic conditions *and their underlying social* determinants.

The key concept of this approach is that concerted action against common health risks and their underlying social determinants will achieve improvements in a range of chronic health conditions more effectively and efficiently than isolated, disease-specific approaches. Adoption of a common risk factor approach is more resource-efficient than a targeted disease-specific approach because:

- most chronic diseases have multiple risk factors
- one risk factor can impact on several diseases

- some risk factors cluster in groups of people
- risk factors can interact—in some instances synergistically—with each other.

The common risk factor approach provides a rationale for developing multi-sectoral healthy alliances between health professionals, statutory, voluntary and commercial bodies and the general public. It recognises that engendering lasting changes in individual "lifestyle" behaviours requires supportive social, economic and political environments.

Common Risk Factors for Oral Health

Oral disease is the most widespread chronic disease, despite being highly preventable. The common risk factors that oral disease shares with other chronic diseases/conditions are:

- **Diet**
  Risk factor for dental caries, coronary heart disease, stroke, diabetes, cancers, obesity
- **Tobacco smoking/chewing**
  Risk factor for oral and other cancers, periodontal disease, coronary heart disease, stroke, respiratory diseases, diabetes
- **Alcohol consumption**
  Risk factor for oral and other cancers, cardiovascular disease, liver cirrhosis, trauma
- **Hygiene**
  Risk factor for periodontal disease and other bacterial and inflammatory conditions
- **Injuries**
  Risk factor for trauma, including dental trauma.
- **Control & Stress**
  Risk factors for periodontal disease and cardiovascular disease

- **Socio-economic status**
  Independent risk factor as well as underlying determinant of other risk factors.

Food Choices and Modern Diet and Dental Caries

Diet is a risk factor for dental caries, coronary heart disease, stroke, diabetes, cancers and obesity.

Diet—the foods and drinks we consume to nourish our body—and our eating habits have an important influence on our health and well-being. A good diet provides the body with the appropriate quantity and quality of nutrients it requires to sustain health. Deficiency diseases such as anaemia and osteoporosis result from the inadequate intake of essential specific nutrients (undernutrition). Overeating or excessive intake of nutrients (over-nutrition) leads to obesity, a recognised major health risk factor.

The oral health message to restrict consumption of foods/drinks containing added sugars to mealtimes complements the healthy heart message to reduce consumption of foods high in oils and fats.

Studies also show that eating more fruits and vegetables can have a protective influence against cancers and systemic inflammatory (including periodontal) diseases.

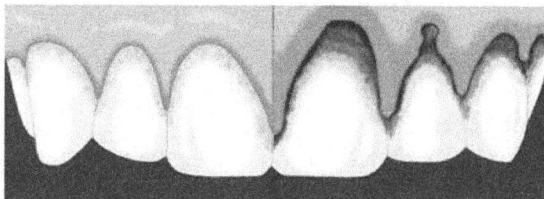

Dental Plaque   Tartar

Dental plaque is a mixture of germs, acid and a sticky substance that continues to grow and becomes hard after a time. As the plaque becomes hard it attaches to teeth very quickly, becoming tartar and usually requires a visit to the dentist to be removed. Tartar becomes calculus, which needs to be scraped off manually.

Signs of plaque: it's not visible normally by visual inspection but, rather, is indicated by bad breath, dental caries, gingival infection and bleeding gums. Usually to see plaque you need disclosing tablets, which discolours plaque. These can be acquired at drugs stores.

Plaque is the main instigator of dental caries and gum problems. Poor gum conditions are associated with many other medical problems from low birth weight, to blood sugar problems and even heart disease (NIH). Dental plaque is not the same as bloodstream plaque and is not related to it.

Dental plaque causes gingivitis, which is not a painful condition, however if your gums bleed on brushing, you most likely have gum problems. In adults this can lead to bone loss around the teeth, in children, this is usually not the case, but it does lead to DC.

So, soft plaque can be removed by twice daily brushing, tartar needs to be removed by dental polishing and calculus is scraped off by dental hygienist. The purpose of a dental preventive program is to control and minimize dental plaque.

[7] http://www.parents.com/baby/health/baby-teeth/cavities/

[8] http://www.medicinenet.com/cavities/article.htm#
what_are_cavities

Chapter 3
The Importance of Prevention

Why Prevention is the Cheapest and Best Treatment

The most important factor in ECC (early childhood caries) is nutrition, or more precisely, the timing of nutrition. Once the primary teeth have erupted and the child continues to feed at will during the night, whether by bottle or by breast feeding, it may lead to severe and rapidly progressing DC, even if you brush the teeth adequately. So the rule is that after the teeth erupt, the child should be given nothing but plain water at night. Human milk is the best for infant nutrition and is not usually associated with ECC. Of course, it may be implicated with frequent night feeding. Fruit juices usually have high sugar content, and the child should get no more than four to six oz/day from a cup (recommendation from American Academy of Pediatricians), night feeding of juices puts the child at greater risk of getting ECC. It also makes sense that frequency and type of snacking can increase the risk of DC.

However, this is not the place for a discussion on nutrition, as there are many cultural, economic and social factors that I cannot address here. The issue is too complex and should be taken up with your dentist if he/she feels qualified.

Changing diet is more difficult to treat and assess and needs full nutritional guidance. However, most nutritionists are not familiar with the effect of different types of nutrition on DC. But it is simple, really, the more frequently the child snacks, and the more sugar-laden the snack, the more likely he or she is to get DC. And as night feeding at will for children who get their first teeth at about one year old will produce DC very quickly the cheapest and best dental treatment is prevention.

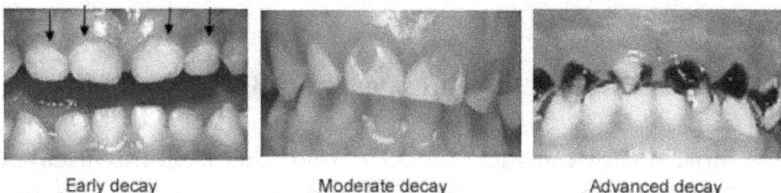

| Early decay | Moderate decay | Advanced decay |

The Importance of Early Dental Caries Assessment

The ideal time for first time assessment is at about one year of age and before any active DC is observed. Assessment must be done by a competent individual: physicians and pediatricians do not have much training and experience in dental and oral development, and many general dentists are not interested in working with young children, or they have little experience in doing so.

No, the best choice for initial assessment is a pediatric dentist and his staff, all of whom are trained and knowledgeable in handling infants and young kids. Many dental hygienists and dentists also lack experience with infants. In fact I have seen many infants who have already been to a dental hygienist because they were not familiar with the proper needs for infants . The brushing technique for adults and young children are very different, as young kids do not have the manual dexterity to brush as an adult, and mouths are smaller and it's more difficult to access all areas of the mouth.

Do not wait for signs of DC, since it is a disease that spreads quickly. Any sign of DC means that many more teeth are already at risk but are not yet showing signs of tooth decay. Dental caries is not only a tooth problem. It can cause gum inflammation and gingivitis as well. Sadly, none of these problems cause pain at an early age; pain is a late symptom and appears only after extensive damage has already been done.

Assessment needs to be done periodically, as situations change and the child or teenager enters a more caries prone time. Also, once you have dental caries you are more prone to get them in the future, thus prevention is optimal.

Note: It is especially important to be vigilant with kids with special needs—they have problems of a medical, physical or developmental nature already, but dental problems can be prevented.

The Main Factors in Prevention are Diet, Nutrition, and Proper Oral Hygiene

Diet and Nutrition

Your body is a complex machine. The foods you choose and how often you eat them can affect your general health and the health of your teeth and gums, too. If you consume too many sugar-filled sodas, sweetened fruit drinks or non-nutritious snacks, you could be at risk for tooth decay. Tooth decay is the single most common chronic childhood disease, but the good news is that it is entirely preventable.

Tooth decay happens when plaque comes into contact with sugar in the mouth causing acid to attack the teeth.

Foods that contain sugars of any kind can contribute to tooth decay. To control the amount of sugar you eat, read the nutrition facts and ingredient labels on foods and beverages and choose options that are lowest in sugar. Common sources of sugar in the diet include soft drinks, candy, cookies and pastries. Your physician or a registered dietitian can also provide suggestions for eating a nutritious diet. For example, if your diet lacks certain nutrients, it may be more difficult for tissues in your mouth to resist infection. This may contribute to gum disease. Severe gum disease is a major cause of tooth loss in adults. Many researchers believe that the disease progresses faster and is potentially more severe in people with poor nutrition.

To learn what foods are best for you, visit ChooseMyPlate.gov, a website from the Center for Nutrition Policy and Promotion, an agency of U.S. Department of Agriculture. The site contains dietary recommendations for children and adults based on their levels of physical activity.

Wise choices

For healthy living and for healthy teeth and gums, think before you eat and drink. It's not only what you eat but when you eat that can affect your dental health. Eat a balanced diet and limit between-meal snacks. If you are on a special diet, keep your physician's advice in mind when choosing foods.

For good dental health, keep these tips in mind when choosing your meals and snacks:

- Drink plenty of water.
- Eat a variety of foods from each of the five major food groups, including:
  o   whole grains
  o   fruits

o vegetables
o lean sources of protein such as lean beef, skinless poultry and fish; and dry beans, peas and other legumes
o low-fat and fat-free dairy foods

Limit the number of snacks you eat. If you do snack, choose something that is healthy like fruit or vegetables or a piece of cheese. Foods that are eaten as part of a meal cause less harm to teeth than eating lots of snacks throughout the day, because more saliva is released during a meal. Saliva helps wash foods from the mouth and lessens the effects of acids, which can harm teeth and cause cavities.

For good dental health, always remember to brush twice a day with fluoride toothpaste that has the American Dental Association Seal of Acceptance, floss daily and visit your dentist regularly. With regular dental care, your dentist can help prevent oral problems from occurring in the first place and catch those that do occur in the early stages, while they are easy to treat.[9]

Creating Awareness of the Dental Home

Another part of prevention is the establishment of the "dental home." The concept of the dental home is derived from the American Academy of Pediatrics concept of the "medical home." The American Academy of Pediatrics states, "the medical care of infants, children, and adolescents ideally should be accessible, continuous, comprehensive, family centered, coordinated, compassionate, and culturally effective. It should be delivered or directed by well-trained physicians who provide primary care and help to manage and facilitate essentially all aspects of pediatric care."

Pediatric primary dental care needs to be delivered in a similar manner. The dental home is a specialized primary dental care provider within the philosophical complex of the medical home. In order to establish a dental home; it is important to meet the parents/ prospective parents early. Gynecologists, pediatricians, and family physicians come in contact with them much before a dentist. He must establish communication with them such that effective and timely referrals are made to the pediatric dentist. Also, schools and pre-school day care centers can be informed about the dental home.

A notice such as—"Do you know you can benefit your child's teeth and oral health by starting preventive dental care *before* child-birth?"—can attract the attention of prospective parents if put in a gynecologist's office. Similarly, the following messages can be displayed in hospitals and clinics of pediatricians, gynecologists and all other pediatric health care professionals:

First Visit by the First Birthday. A child should visit the pediatric dentist within six months of the eruption of the first tooth or by age one. Early examination and preventive care will protect your child's smile now and in the future.

Dental problems can begin early. A big concern is the Early Childhood Caries (also known as baby bottle tooth decay or nursing caries). Children risk severe decay from using a bottle during night feeding.

The earlier the dental visit, the better the chance of preventing dental problems. Children with healthy teeth chew food easily, are better able to learn to speak clearly and smile with confidence. Start children now on a lifetime of good dental habits.

Encourage children to drink from a cup as they approach their first birthday. Children should not fall asleep with a bottle. At-will, night time breast-feeding should be avoided after the first primary teeth begin to erupt. Drinking juice from a bottle should be avoided. When juice is offered, it should be in a cup.

Children should be weaned from the bottle at 12-14 months of age.

Thumb sucking is perfectly normal for infants; most stop by the age of two but it should be discouraged after age four. Prolonged thumb sucking can create crowded, crooked teeth or bite problems. Dentists can suggest ways to address a prolonged thumb sucking habit.

Never dip a pacifier into honey or anything sweet before giving it to a baby, and limit the frequency of snacking, which can increase a child's risk of developing cavities.

Parents should ensure that young children use an appropriate size toothbrush with a small brushing surface and only a pea-sized amount of fluoride toothpaste at each brushing. Young children should always be supervised while brushing and taught to spit out rather than swallow the toothpaste. Unless advised to do so by a dentist or other health professionals, parents should not use fluoride toothpaste for children less than two years of age.

Children who drink primarily bottled water may not be getting the fluoride they need.

From six months to age three, children may have sore gums when teeth erupt. Many children like a clean teething ring, cool spoon, or cold wet washcloth. Some parents prefer a chilled ring; others simply rub the baby's gums with a clean finger.

Parents and caregivers need to take care of their own teeth so that cavity-causing bacteria are not as easily transmitted to children. Don't clean pacifiers and eating utensils with your own mouth before giving them to children. That can also transmit adults' bacteria to children.

Basic Preventative Strategies

Historically, the approach to preventing the development of dental caries has been to establish and maintain good oral hygiene, optimize systemic and topical fluoride exposure, and eliminate prolonged exposure to simple sugars in the diet. The success of this age-old approach is also the foundation for the ideal standard of establishment of the dental home by one year of age as endorsed by; the American Dental Association; the American Academy of Pediatric Dentistry; supporting organizations of Bright Futures and numerous other children's health organizations.

Dental caries typically results from diet-mediated shifts in dental bacterial populations that favor acidogenic-aciduric (cariogenic) organisms. The judicious optimization of diet, fluoride intake, and hygiene reverses the aciduric shift, resulting in fewer cariogenic flora and decreased rates of caries. Clinical observations suggest that aciduric shifts are often associated with pregnancy, with return to pre-pregnancy cariogenic-benign flora ratio occurring on the same timeline as the colonization of the infant with dental flora (6 to 30 months of age). The overall strategy is to lower the numbers of cariogenic bacteria in the mother's mouth and delay colonization as long as possible (avoid sharing of spoons, orally cleansing pacifiers, etc).

Tooth decay is a disease that is, by and large, preventable. Because of how it is caused and when it begins however, steps to prevent it ideally should begin prenatally with pregnant women and continue with the mother and young child, beginning when the infant is approximately six months of age. The primary thrust of early risk assessment is to screen for parent-infant groups who are at risk of early childhood dental caries and would benefit from early aggressive intervention. The ultimate goal of early assessment is the timely delivery of educational information to populations at high risk of caries to avoid the need for later surgical intervention.

Oral Health Risk Assessment

Every child should begin to receive oral health risk assessments by a Pediatric Dentist by 1 year of age. The Caries Risk Assessment Tool (provided and continually updated by the American Academy of Pediatric Dentistry and available at http://www. aapd.org/members/referencemanual/pdfs/02-03/ Caries%20Risk%20Assess.pdf) can be used to determine the relative risk of caries of the patient. In the case of the very young patient, a risk assessment to identify parents (usually mothers) and infants with a high predisposition to caries can easily be performed by taking a simple dental history from a new mother. Questions directed at dietary practices, fluoride exposure, oral hygiene, utilization of dental services, and the number and location of the mother's dental fillings can give a relative indication of the mother's baseline decay potential. Frequent sugar intake, low fluoride exposure, poor oral hygiene practices, infrequent utilization of dental services and/or active decay and/or multiple dental fillings in multiple quadrants of the mouth indicates a high caries risk in the mother. Because the dental history of the mother has a direct correlation to that of her infant, it is justifiable and appropriate for the pediatrician to garner permission to examine the mother's dentition and gingival tissues. Additionally, clinical observations suggest that second and third infants tend to be colonized earlier, when the mother's cariogenic flora is at a higher level. Therefore, the later-order offspring of a mother with mildly to moderately high caries rate may be at higher risk of caries than are offspring born earlier. Unfortunately, the lack of accessible longitudinal dental databases has not yet allowed these observations to be epidemiologically confirmed.

Risk Groups for Dental Caries

The caries risk potential of an infant can be determined by the use of the Caries Risk Assessment Tool. However, even the most judiciously designed and implemented caries risk assessment tool can fail to identify all infants at risk of early childhood dental caries. If an infant is assessed to be within one of the following risk groups, the care requirements would be significant and surgically invasive. Therefore, these infants should be referred to a Pediatric Dentist as early as six months of age and no later than six months after the first tooth erupts or 12 months of age (whichever comes first) for establishment of a dental home. The risk groups mentioned include children with special health care needs; of mothers with a high caries rate; with demonstrable caries, plaque, demineralization, and/or staining; who sleep with a bottle or breastfeed throughout the night; in families of low socioeconomic status; and later-order offspring. However, despite all efforts to predict children at high risk of caries, patients can and do fall outside statistical expectations. In these cases, the mother may not be the colonization source of the child's dental flora instead, the dietary intake of simple carbohydrates may be extremely high, or other uncontrollable factors may combine to place the patient at risk of caries. Therefore, screening for risk of caries in the parent and patient coupled with oral health counseling, although a feasible and equitable approach to early childhood caries control, is not a substitute for early establishment of the dental home. Whenever possible, the ideal approach to early childhood caries prevention and management is the early establishment of a dental home.

Oral Health Risk Assessment and the Dental Home

Six months after the first tooth erupts, or by 12 months of age, the child's dental home should be established and provide an opportunity to implement preventive dental health habits that meet each child's unique needs and keep the child free from dental or oral disease. The dental home should be expected to provide:

- an accurate risk assessment for dental diseases and conditions;
- an individualized preventive dental health program based on the risk assessment;
- a plan for emergency dental trauma;
- anticipatory guidance about growth and development issues (ie, teething, digit or pacifier habits, and feeding practices);
- comprehensive dental care in accordance with accepted guidelines and periodicity schedules for pediatric dental health;
- information about proper care of the child's teeth and gingival tissues;
- information regarding proper nutrition and dietary practices; and
- referrals to other dental specialists, such as endodontists, oral surgeons, orthodontists, and periodontists, when care cannot be provided directly within the dental home.

Anticipatory Guidance and Parent and Patient Education

General anticipatory guidance for the mother (or other intimate caregiver) before and during the colonization process should include the following:

Caries removal—parents should be referred to a dentist for an examination and restoration of all active decay as soon as feasible.
Delay of colonization—mothers should be educated to prevent early colonization of dental flora in their infants by avoiding sharing of utensils (ie, shared spoons, cleaning a dropped pacifier with their saliva, etc).
Diet—the parent should be instructed to consume fruit juices only at meals and to avoid all carbonated beverages during the first 30 months of the infant's life.
Fluoride—the parent should be instructed to use a fluoride toothpaste approved by the American Dental Association.
Oral hygiene—the parent should be instructed to brush thoroughly twice daily (morning and evening) and to floss at least once every day.
Oral hygiene—the parent should begin to brush the child's teeth as soon as they erupt (twice daily, morning and evening) and floss between the child's teeth once every day as soon as teeth contact one another.

Recommendations

The infectious and transmissible nature of bacteria that cause early childhood caries and methods of oral health risk assessment, anticipatory guidance, and early intervention, should be included in the curriculum of all pediatric medical residency programs and postgraduate continuing medical education curricula at an appropriate time. Early childhood caries is an infectious and preventable disease that is vertically transmitted from mothers or other intimate caregivers to infants. All health care professionals who serve mothers and infants should integrate parent and caregiver education into their practices that instruct effective methods of prevention of early childhood caries. Pediatricians, family practitioners, and pediatric nurse practitioners and physician assistants should be trained to perform an oral health risk assessment on all children by six months of age to identify known risk factors for early childhood dental caries. They should also support the concept of the identification of a dental home as an ideal for all children in the early toddler years. Infants identified as having significant risk of caries or assessed to be within one of the risk groups listed in this statement should be entered into an aggressive anticipatory guidance and intervention program provided by a dentist between 6 and 12 months of age. And finally, every child should begin to receive oral health risk assessments by six months of age from a pediatrician or a qualified pediatric health care professional.

Summary

Early childhood dental caries emerges within all cultural and economic pediatric populations however, it approaches near epidemic proportions in populations with low socioeconomic status. Dental caries is an infectious disease usually passed from mother to child from generation to generation. Judicious optimization of diet, fluoride intake, and hygiene can decrease bacterial levels of specific organisms responsible for dental caries residing within normal dental flora. Decreasing the levels of cariogenic flora in the mother before and during the colonization process coupled with counseling directed toward optimal practices of diet, oral hygiene, and fluoride exposure can significantly and positively impact the child's predisposition to early childhood caries. Patients who have been determined to be at risk of development of dental caries or who fall into recognized risk groups should be directed to establish a dental home six months after the first tooth erupts or by one year of age (whichever comes first). The ideal deterrence to early childhood caries is the establishment of the dental home when indicated by the unique needs of the child. Although not always feasible because of manpower and participation issues, best practice dictates that all patients should have a comprehensive dental examination by a dentist in the early toddler years.[10]

The Importance of Proper Tooth Brushing

You have been brushing your teeth for most of your life, but are you really brushing teeth properly? The importance of brushing teeth properly is often overlooked, but it's an important part of keeping your teeth and gums healthy.

Most of us don't really pay attention when we're brushing. Instead, you may brush distractedly while thinking about your day, to-do lists or your weekend plans. While brushing your teeth properly isn't rocket science, it does require a conscious effort to make sure it's done right and for maximum effect.

Tips on Brushing Teeth Properly

The most common pitfall that keeps people from brushing teeth properly is that they don't brush for long enough. Most dentists recommend brushing for two to three minutes, spending at least 30 seconds on each "quadrant" of your mouth. Brushing teeth properly means taking care to reach every tooth as well as every surface of every tooth. Don't forget your tongue. The tongue harbors a multitude of bacteria, particularly those that contribute to oral malodor. You can use a regular brush or a tongue scraper. In fact, many toothbrushes now feature textured tongue cleaners. One example is the Oral-B CrossAction Pro-Health Toothbrush. By brushing teeth properly, you can help keep your mouth and teeth in good health for years to come.

Although there are other modalities such as flossing, rinsing mouth with mouthwash and water picks, these are just adjunct services that are not important if the teeth have not been thoroughly brushed. Although brushing teeth is important, it is important only if done effectively, so that teeth are clean and dental plaque removed daily. Many people come in and are perplexed that their children have DC even though they brush their teeth three times a day. The importance of brushing is that it removes the dental plaque and if not, it is useless. Most of the time parents should be brushing teeth of preschoolers. Children do not have the manual dexterity or patience to brush teeth well, or remove plaque. Most parents do not brush hard enough or long enough to do an effective job. A toothbrush is not a magic wand that if you wave it around in your mouth for 20 seconds removes plaque, thus the importance of brushing is that each tooth surface is reached, that enough time is spent brushing, and that it is done firmly. If these efforts are not effective, DC will result in time. Many parents let children brush teeth on their own, without supervision, again not an effective way to remove dental plaque, so do not be surprised that child gets tooth decay. If you would not have your child clean your house, why do you think they will be able to clean their teeth properly? If your house cannot be cleaned in 10 minutes, what makes you think you can clean your teeth and mouth in 10 seconds? Part of dental assessment is effectiveness of your child's brushing and cleaning and oral hygiene habits.

The reason you will get tooth decay, even though you brush your child's teeth three times daily, is you do not get the plaque off daily, the plaque changes in nature; when it first forms it is soft, and can be removed by manual brushing; after a day or two it becomes firmly attached to the teeth and cannot be removed anymore by simple tooth brushing, but will now stay and accumulate, until removed professionally by dentist and hygienist. Thus daily effective brushing is mandatory and periodic assessments and cleaning is important. This should be done by a pediatric dentist or dentist who treats children routinely, as brushing technique is different than for an adult, and many dentists and hygienists are not aware of this (if they do not treat kids daily).

For one to two year-olds let the child play with a toothbrush (TB), but parents must brush his/her teeth for about one minute two times daily; in the morning, after breakfast and at night before going to sleep, after the last feeding. Use scrubbing technique, back and forth, brush firmly using a small soft bristle toothbrush. The child may struggle and not be cooperative, and may cry, but firm brushing with a gentle toothbrush is not painful. A slight amount of bleeding (pink tb) is a sign of poor oral hygiene and demands more vigorous technique. If bleeding persists after seven days of brushing, or you think that the child is having pain on brushing, a dental assessment should be done.

Flossing

People have all sorts of excuses for not flossing their teeth.

You don't floss so much to remove food from the teeth, you do it to get rid of plaque, the bacterial film that forms between teeth and along your gum line. Doing so daily prevents gum disease and tooth loss. Everyone gets plaque, and it can only be removed by flossing or a deep cleaning from your dentist.

Flossing is "the most difficult personal grooming activity there is," says Samuel B. Low, DDS, a professor at the University of

Florida and past president of the American Academy of Periodontology. But it's one of the most important to learn.

The American Dental Association gives these tips for flossing right: Use 18 inches of floss. Wrap most of it around the middle finger of one hand, the rest around your other middle finger. Grasp the string tightly between your thumb and forefinger, and use a rubbing motion to guide it between teeth. When the floss reaches the gum line, form a C to follow the shape of the tooth. Hold the strand firmly against the tooth, and move it gently up and down. Repeat with the other tooth, and then repeat the entire process with the rest of your teeth. Use fresh sections of floss as you go. Don't forget the back of your last molars. "By far, most gum disease and most decay occurs in the back teeth," Low says. If you have trouble reaching the back of your mouth, ask your dentist about using one of these tools: plastic, disposable, Y-shaped flossers that allow for extra reach; small, round brushes; pointed, rubber tips; or wooden or plastic pics (called interdental cleaners). A child will need your help to floss until he's about 11 years old. Kids should start to floss as soon as they have two teeth that touch.[11]

Preventive Programs That Are Age Specific

Brushing for Infants

Brushing for a child one to three years-old should happen twice daily, one at morning, after breakfast, or feeding, the second time just before going to sleep. If the child is difficult, brushing once daily is adequate—if done well. The purpose is to ingrain good oral hygiene habits at a young age, and to remove plague daily. Many infants like brushing, but some do not. Be prepared for a struggle at the beginning. Although the child may struggle and fight and even cry, be aware you are not hurting your child if brushing properly, but you must persist to start good habits and effective oral hygiene. Too many parents give up early on proper brushing because it is such a fight, and they do not want to upset their kids. However, what would you do if your child persists in playing in the middle of the road? You know this is dangerous and you would stop them however many times it took for them to get the message. DC is dangerous and requires the same due diligence as in the former example.

Many times when you start brushing firmly, you will notice that your child's gums bleed on brushing, and since the child is crying and fighting, you presume you are hurting the child, and you stop brushing, or you brush less firmly. This is exactly wrong. Most of the time a child's gums bleed because they have gingivitis, due to lack of good oral hygiene. So if you are not brushing properly, and removing dental plaque, it accumulates and gives off poisons and toxins that inflame the gums and make them bleed on brushing. Thus bleeding gums on brushing is a sign that teeth are not clean, and brushing is not effective, or not being done. In such instances, you need to do the exact opposite of what you have been doing. The teeth need to be brushed firmly, especially in the bleeding area, and if caught early, after three-four days of adequate brushing, the gums will stop bleeding on their own and gingivitis will heal with no need for medications, or antibiotics.

If you are brushing well and bleeding persists, then you need to get this checked by your pediatric dentist as there may be other problems causing the bleeding. Also, if gums bleed profusely after two-three days of proper brushing, bring your child to a pediatric dentist for a full assessment to rule out any medical conditions.

Another reason to attack plaque in bleeding areas is that the plaque that causes gingivitis will eventually cause DC. If your child already has DC, it may be painful to brush in these areas, and child will continue to struggle. Note: if a child does have pain on brushing, this is a sign that treatment will be necessary. Some things to remember about brushing: if you can brush only once, just before going to sleep is the best time; you do not need to brush after every meal or feeding; pick up a soft toothbrush, one with a small head, so that you can reach the back areas of the mouth; use a scrub, back and forth technique not the adult roll technique, as this is too difficult and not as effective in cleaning. There is no need to floss, as kids have a short attention span and trying to floss is difficult —by the time you get to brushing all the child's good behavior is used up.

Three Year-old Brushing and Prevention

By three years of age all baby teeth have erupted, and the child has become more cavity prone because molars have deep grooves and collect food and plaque. The back teeth are also more difficult to get at with a TB.

When molars first come in there is space between teeth and the area is self-cleaning, but as the child and jaws develop, the space between the teeth is eliminated and they become more prone to getting DC. Therefore, cleaning must be more effective. This is the ideal time to add a fluoride (FL) toothpaste (TP), as FL is effective in preventing flat surface DC between teeth. Use a smudge, or pea sized dab of TP when brushing twice a day. Most children this age are not yet spitting but swallowing a small amount of TP is not harmful. Note: Children's TP is sweet tasting, so keep the tube out of the reach of children, so they do not swallow the whole tube at once.

While brushing, you must use a firm technique, making sure to reach back of molars. If the child is reluctant, you must still be firm and continue. If this is not possible, have an oral assessment done as they may have a condition that causes pain on eating and brushing. Example: primary herpes is a painful disease of mouth with many small blisters, making brushing and eating very difficult. It is a viral infection that lasts about 7-10 days.

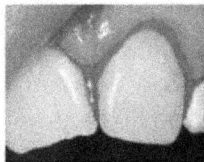

Periodic bleeding gums shows lack of good hygiene. You need to brush harder, longer, and get to difficult areas. If bleeding persists, an oral assessment is necessary to find the cause—from primary herpes to gingivitis to hemophilia or other medical conditions.

Many kids are reluctant to have parents brush. They want to do it themselves. If this is the case, let them brush, and then finish it for them. They are not yet effective brushers, but they do need to start good habits early in life.

Remember, if your child complains of pain, it may be due to DC starting (it is easy to miss). Take your child in for an assessment. With a child this age, after proper brushing, you may floss to remove food caught between teeth. As mentioned previously, flossing is best way to prevent cavities between teeth and should be done with proper brushing and a FL TP.

Five Year-old Brushing and Prevention

At this age, the child's jaws are developing and growing to accommodate permanent molars. These teeth erupt behind baby molars and parents may be unaware because there is no pain or discomfort in eruption and no teeth fall out here. In order to access the back molars properly, you should brush the teeth with the mouth closed. If you open widely, the cheeks get in the way and you cannot adequately clean the teeth. A good hygienist will be able to show you how to do this. Note: using an adult brushing technique will not do an adequate job of cleaning.

You will still need a TB with a small head in order to adequately get to difficult to reach areas. Gagging on brushing is a sign that child does not want to have his or her teeth brushed. There are a number of things that could be behind this behavior: if there is DC, then the area could be painful or the TP may have a burning sensation (in which case try brushing without TP). Bottom line - If your child remains reluctant, get a dental assessment.

The TP you should be using at this age is a child TP, not an infant TP which has no FL. Use an amount about the size of a pea. You should be aware that some kids have soft teeth (cavity prone and sensitive to brushing and to cold). These teeth need an immediate assessment, as they will decay much earlier than normal teeth.

At this age, the lower front teeth are getting loose, to let permanent incisors erupt. The lower front teeth also become mobile, and some finicky kids refuse to brush in this area, as it may be uncomfortable, or child may be scared to loosen teeth further. This is easily seen as most of mouth is clean, except in area of lose teeth. If lose teeth are really painful and child will not brush or chew in this area, the offending teeth should be extracted. This will allow the child to function properly and to brush properly.

Parents must remember that brushing needs to be effective. If you feel your child is not brushing properly, then you must do it for him or her. Because children have such a short attention span, you should concentrate on effective brushing for two-three minutes, flossing the molars only if the child remains co-operative. The ideal times to brush are right after breakfast and just before going to sleep. Remember, pink toothbrush bristles is a sign of gingivitis, and improper brushing in that area.

8- 12 Year-old Brushing and Prevention

An 8-12 year-old child will have anywhere from 12-28 permanent teeth. Brushing must be more effective especially in the area of molars, as teeth that are newly erupted are more cavity-prone and need FL to help them prevent DC. Children with loose teeth may be more reluctant to brush firmly in these areas and loose teeth can stay that way for many months if not disturbed. Some effective ideas are to brush just before bedtime, spit out TP and not rinse out mouth, as FL will stay on teeth for a prolonged period of time, and be more effective. Also, most kids do not have manual dexterity to do adult tooth brushing techniques, so have them use scrub or circular motions. At this age an electric toothbrush can be very helpful. If the child still will not brush in an area it may be due to those lose baby teeth or DC. An evaluation by a dentist should be done before the erupting permanent teeth decay.

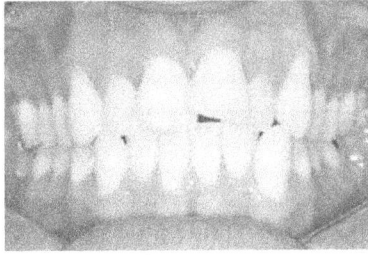

Many children have crowded teeth, making these teeth more difficult to clean and often leading to DC. In these circumstances dental assessment is mandatory.

Children with braces should use an electric toothbrush, as it is much more difficult to do an effective job of brushing and removing plaque from around each bracket. It is useful to remember that if your child is being seen by an orthodontist, he or she will not really check for tooth decay, and by the time he/she notices any DC it may already be quite large and need extensive treatment. Also, children with braces who do not brush well will find that when the braces are removed there is a white spotting of the teeth, which is in fact a decalcification and start of DC.

12- 18 Year-old Brushing and Prevention

These children should be able to brush by themselves unsupervised for two-three minutes two times per day, morning and night. Adult brushing technique should now be used, as a scrub and circular technique can cause gum recession, and tooth sensitivity. This is an ideal time to introduce flossing after brushing. An electric toothbrush is always helpful to get teeth clean and prevent tartar build up. Remember that areas where teeth are crowded or crooked need special attention.

It is important to prevent DC at this stage because large DC, even if filled, may lead to replacement fillings at a later date as fillings may break or the teeth may break, leading to more complex treatment such as crowns and possible root canal treatment to retain teeth.

If you can remain caries free by the age of 18, you will be unlikely to get DC in the future. But remember, even if you do not get DC by 18 yr., if brushing is inadequate it will lead to gingivitis, which is a precursor to periodontitis, which will eventually also lead to tooth loss. Signs of gingivitis are bleeding gums on brushing. Periodontitis can only be evaluated by a dentist in the initial stages when it is easily treatable and reversible. If necessary a referral to a gum specialist may be required.

At this age, if a patient is deemed caries prone, the adjunct of a FL mouth rinse may be recommended. A FL mouth rinse is a good idea, and is one of the best ways to prevent DC between teeth if brushing is being done effectively. I do not advise mouth rinses for children younger than 12 years of age, as they might swallow the rinse or not use it effectively.

Prevention and the Special Needs Child

Children with special needs, whether due to physical, medical or mental conditions, may present a dental challenge. There is a wide range of conditions from mild and barely noticeable, to complete lack of co-operation for basic assessment and treatment. Many dentists are intimidated by special needs children and will not treat them. Pediatric dentists are in a unique position with special training to meet the dental needs of all special needs kids, and usually have a hospital affiliation to do any necessary treatment beyond routine dental preventive care.

Some children with special needs do not communicate well, and may be in pain, but not be able to communicate their problems. These kids have all sorts of challenges, but most dental problems can be prevented by an early and adequate dental assessment followed up by a routinely monitored, preventive dental program.

Oral hygiene should not be neglected, and although not optimum, you have to do the best you can. There will be good days and bad days, and as long as there are more good days than bad days do not get frustrated. If they can tolerate an electric toothbrush, it will help to do an effective job. You can use FL toothpaste but only a small amount, the size of a pea, as they will swallow TP. If you can complete brushing, flossing should be done as well. I do not recommend mouth rinse. Also, I cannot stress enough the importance of regular recall, so as not to let problems fester and deteriorate. Many of these kids do quite well on good, routine, preventive programs. Over time, most will get to know the staff and actually enjoy their dental outing.

Routine Recall Exams

The recommended interval between oral health reviews should be determined specifically for each patient, and tailored to meet his or her needs, on the basis of an assessment of disease levels and risk of or from dental disease. This assessment should integrate the evidence presented in this guideline with the clinical judgement and expertise of the dental team, and should be discussed with the patient. During an oral health review, the dental team (led by the dentist) should ensure that comprehensive histories are taken, examinations are conducted and initial preventive advice is given. This will allow the dental team and the patient (and/or his or her parent, guardian or caregiver) to discuss, where appropriate:

- the effects of oral hygiene, diet, fluoride use, tobacco and alcohol on oral health;
- the risk factors that may influence the patient's oral health, and their implications for deciding the appropriate recall interval;
- the outcome of previous care episodes and the suitability of previously recommended intervals;
- the patient's ability or desire to visit the dentist at the recommended interval; and
- the financial costs to the patient of having the oral health review and any subsequent treatments.

The interval before the next oral health review should be chosen, either at the end of an oral health review if no further treatment is indicated, or on completion of a specific treatment journey. The recommended shortest and longest intervals between oral health reviews are as follows: The shortest interval between oral health reviews for all patients should be three months. The longest interval between oral health reviews for patients younger than 18 years should be 12 months. The longest interval between oral health reviews for patients aged 18 years and older should be 24 months. The dentist should discuss the recommended recall interval with the patient and record this interval, and the patient's agreement or disagreement with it, in the current record-keeping system.

The recall interval should be reviewed again at the next oral health visit, in order to learn from the patient's responses to the oral care provided and the health outcomes achieved. This feedback and the findings of the oral health review should be used to adjust the next recall interval chosen. Patients should be informed that their recommended recall interval may vary over time.

What Happens When Prevention Does Not Work?

Acute Dental Trauma Prevention

Facial trauma that results in fractured, displaced, or lost teeth can have significant negative functional, esthetic, and psychological effects on children. Dentists and physicians should collaborate to educate the public about prevention and treatment of traumatic injuries to the oral and maxillofacial region. The greatest incidence of trauma to the primary teeth occurs at two to three years of age, when motor coordination is developing. The most common injuries to permanent teeth occur because of falls, followed by traffic accidents, violence, and sports. All sporting activities have an associated risk of orofacial injuries due to falls, collisions, and contact with hard surfaces. The AAPD encourages the use of protective gear, including mouth guards, which help distribute forces of impact, thereby reducing the risk of severe injury. Dental injuries could have improved outcomes if the public were aware of first-aid measures and the need to seek immediate treatment. Because optimal treatment results follow immediate assessment and care, dentists have an ethical obligation to ensure that reasonable arrangements for emergency dental care are available. The history, circumstances of the injury, pattern of trauma, and behavior of the child and/or caregiver are important in distinguishing non-abusive injuries from abuse. Practitioners have the responsibility to recognize, differentiate, and either appropriately manage or refer children with acute oral traumatic injuries, as dictated by the complexity of the injury and the individual clinician's training, knowledge, and experience. Compromised airway, neurological manifestations (eg, altered orientation), hemorrhage, nausea/vomiting, or suspected loss of consciousness requires further evaluation by a physician. To efficiently determine the extent of injury and correctly diagnose injuries to the teeth, periodontium, and associated structures, a systematic approach to the traumatized child is essential. Assessment includes a thorough medical and dental history, clinical and radiographic examination, and additional tests such as palpation, percussion, sensitivity, and mobility evaluation. Intraoral radiography is useful for the evaluation of dentoalveolar trauma. If the area of concern extends beyond the dentoalveolar complex, extraoral imaging may be indicated. Treatment planning takes into consideration the patient's health status and developmental status, as well as extent of injuries. Advanced behavior guidance techniques or an appropriate referral may be necessary to ensure that proper diagnosis and care are given. All relevant diagnostic information, treatment, and recommended follow-up care should be documented in the patient's record. A standardized trauma form can guide the practitioner's clinical assessment and provide a way to record the essential aspects of care in an organized and consistent manner.

Insurance Coverage and Prevention

Why does my dental plan only cover a selection of treatment?
Dental plans are developed to offset some of the costs of treatment and generally include a selection of coverage; they are not developed based on your unique dental care needs, nor do they cover the full range of dental treatment services available. Dental plans are selected by the plan purchaser, usually as part of a group benefits plan. Many plans will cover a range of diagnostic (examination) and preventive services (scaling, polishing). Such services are common to all patients and aid in the prevention of dental disease. Bear in mind that these plans may also have limits on the amount or frequency of services and treatment which is not based on what any individual may actually need. Additional treatment services will vary, as will

the percentage of coverage patients receive for treatments covered by the plan.

Why can't my dentist create a treatment plan based on my dental plan coverage?

Your dentist's first obligation is to your health. If you have an issue with your mouth your dentist will present treatment options to meet your oral and overall health needs; your treatment plan is not based on your dental plan coverage. Your dentist can help you to get a pre-determination for treatment to understand what costs may be covered by your dental plan.

It is important to make your treatment decisions based on your health care needs, not based on what your dental plan covers. Speak to your dentist about his or her treatment recommendations and cost estimates along with any consequences in delaying or refusing treatment so you can make an informed choice for your health.

Why doesn't my dentist/dental office know what my plan covers?

There are many dental plan options available. Plan coverage is determined by you and/or your employer. The details of your plan are protected by the *Personal Health Information Privacy and Access Act (PHIPAA)*. While your dentist can help you understand your plan, they do not know the details of your plan and/or any changes that may occur.

It is your responsibility to understand what your plan covers. It is important to be aware of any financial limits and changes to your plan.

Do I need a dental plan?

If you do not benefit from a dental plan provided by your employer you may wish to consider purchasing a private dental plan to help offset some of the costs of care. This is particularly valuable in accessing preventive services.

Many plans include a range of diagnostic (an examination by a dentist) and preventive (scaling, polishing) treatment services, generally covering a higher percentage of the associated costs. Such services can aid in the prevention of dental disease, identify trouble signs early and lead to less complex and costly treatment in the future. In considering a dental plan you may want to determine whether the annual cost of the premiums are preferable to simply budgeting for dental care.

[9]http://www.mouthhealthy.org/en/az-topics/d/diet-and-dental-health

[10]http://pediatrics.aappublications.org/content/111/5/1113.full.pdf

[11]http://www.webmd.com/oral-health/healthy-teeth-14/flossing-floss-sticks

Chapter 4
Dental Treatment for Kids

Why a Pediatric Dentist (cont'd)?

For most people a child is the most precious thing in your life. There is very little you wouldn't do for them. So who should treat your child when it comes to dental matters? The answer is a Pediatric Dentist. Here's why: unlike many local dental offices a pediatric dentist will treat any kid—even those three and under. You see, they are equipped and prepared to handle your child if more than routine work is involved. A regular dentist probably won't be. And as many areas of the country do not have access to pediatric dentists, be sure to get a referral to the doctor nearest to you.

Did you know there have been cases of parents going to clinics and getting dental treatment that they thought was by a specialist but was in fact by a dentist with minimal training and experience? Some of the outcomes have been adverse to say the least—due to inadequate treatment that needs to be done over. And in addition to putting your child through another needless and difficult set of procedures, be aware that dental insurance will not reimburse you for that second treatment , you are on your own. And as if that were not enough, there have also been fatal outcomes from dentists treating kids under sedation when they are not properly trained and when they do not treat kids routinely.

As mentioned previously, the Pediatric Dentist goes back to school for two-three years for additional training. He or she not only learns how to treat teeth, but also studies the multitude of medical conditions that oral health care can cover, always with your child's general health in mind. From special needs kids to developmentally delayed kids; to kids with psychological problems and medical problems; to children with Down's Syndrome, hemophilia and other bleeding disorders; to children with heart murmurs who need special attention; and even to children with physical disabilities who need special dental care, the Pediatric Dentist is trained to deal with every situation that comes to mind.

The plain truth of the matter is that many parents with special needs kids or children with severe medical conditions are overwhelmed and just cope day to day, overlooking oral and dental needs until it is too late and extensive costly treatment is necessary. Additionally, a poor initial dental experience will lead to child being resistant to further treatment, or the parent may be upset and not want to put the child through another bad experience and will thus put off necessary dental treatment.

If your child has had a bad experience, speak to the dentist of possible ways to handle the problem—perhaps referral to another more experienced dentist, or using a different type of sedation. Putting treatment off until a child grows up is not an option, decay will deteriorate the teeth with time and treatment will be more extensive and likely more painful as caries gets close to nerves so that even freezing will not dull all the pain.

In a pediatric dental office not only is the dentist trained to treat all variety of kids but his staff—the dental assistants, the hygienists and the front desk people are also experienced in dealing with children and their dental problems. Other dental offices may need to deal with adults and their needs, and fitting in a difficult or frightened child is not conducive to the child having a good experience. The fact is, many parents take their kids to their personal dentist, and this is fine, but ask him or her ahead of time if they feel comfortable treating your child. And please don't make the mistake of having the child in the operatory during your own dental treatment. I am against this, as the child does not understand what is happening, and even if you are comfortable getting an injection, the child will not see this in a positive light. If you are even the slightest bit apprehensive, your body language will betray you, and the child will not feel comfortable. Conversely, watching a sibling is not good either, because if the child acts up this will also send the wrong message. No, the best way to introduce the child to the dental environment is in a non-confrontational way, as a visit of introduction or an initial exam and observation. Again, ideally, the first visit should be at about one year of age, but no later than three years.

* * *

There is a saying that "You have British teeth," and it's not a compliment. Britain's standards fall behind with respect to those of North America. The following partial piece was adapted from an article in a recent British newspaper and is yet another example of why early prevention with a Pediatric Dentist is crucial. See if you can pick up the difference between what I have recommended and what is recommended by the dentist in the article …

My children Refuse to Brush Their Teeth

Every evening as I get my two year old son Felix ready for bed he will look at me reproachfully, and then run away. I chase after him with pleas and bribes, before resorting to threats about what will happen should he refuse to do as I say. When that, too, fails, I corner him in a headlock, pry his mouth open and force his toothbrush inside. Afterwards there are cross words and tearful recriminations—from me as well as my toddler.

I have always found cleaning my children's teeth an emotionally-charged nightmare, as do millions of other parents. A report last month found that 42 per cent of parents have to force their children (aged up to 11) to brush their teeth, with 80 per cent of youngsters throwing temper tantrums as they do so. *Only a quarter of the 1558 parents surveyed by Aquafresh believe their children are brushing their teeth properly and one in 10 are so demoralised by the process they send their offspring to bed without cleaning them at all.*

But our acquiescence comes at a cost. *A national dental health survey published in May revealed almost half of eight-year-olds have signs of decay in their milk teeth, while a recent report by the Royal College of Surgeons (RCS) found that tooth decay was the most common reason five to nine year olds were admitted to hospital. Nearly 26,000 children in that age group were admitted in 2013-14, an increase of 14 per cent from 2011.*

Professor Nigel Hunt, Dean of the Royal College of Surgeon's dental faculty, was quoted as saying, "The state of our children's teeth has reached [a] "crisis point," adding that, "It is absolutely intolerable that in this day and age, in a civilised country, children are having so many teeth out for decay, which is over 90 per cent preventable."

But substandard brushing and infrequent dentist visits are also to blame for rising child tooth decay, and I am complicit in all three. I find it hard to resist my children's incessant demands for sweet treats, and our fraught tooth brushing sessions usually fall short of the NHS recommended twice daily two minutes. And shamefully, until very recently I had yet to take either child to the dentist. A fear of how they would react was the deterrent. With every passing month I grew more worried that my neglect would lead to lasting dental problems, and retreat further into denial. However, the spate of news stories on the state of our children's teeth jolted me into action, and so it was that one day last month, they were sitting in my dentist's reception awaiting their first check-up.

I tried to build enthusiasm for the visit, but both were nervous. "Are you scared of the dentist, too, Mummy?" asked my daughter, and although I didn't admit as much to her, my own fear has almost certainly exacerbated my children's reluctance. Indeed, research by a US dental insurance company found that over a third of kids were frightened of the dentist and that this was often a learned behaviour, picked up from parents.

Problems with my own teeth have also left me distrustful of NHS dentistry, which I feel has failed me, so I took my children to my dentist, who runs a private practice in North London. He encourages parents to bring their children in from the age of two. "As long as parents are brushing their baby's teeth, I can't see the point of bringing them to the dentist any younger," he says. "It's unnecessary until they have grown around 75 percent of teeth."

But, he warns: "Many parents mistakenly believe that milk teeth don't matter because they are going to fall out anyway. But they act as 'space maintainers' for the permanent teeth that replace them. If a decaying milk tooth has to be removed the 'wrong' tooth may come forward in its place."

After a few minutes of the children riding up and down in the dentist's chair, my daughter was relaxed enough to have her check-up. On the pretence of "counting her teeth" the doctor used a hand-held mirror to inspect her molars as my son looked on. It took a matter of minutes and afterwards the dentist told my delighted daughter (and her mum) that her teeth were "absolutely fine."

My son, however, had by this time hidden in the corner of the room and was resolutely refusing to open his mouth. My dentist was reluctant to force him but after bribes of Spiderman stickers Felix eventually permitted a brief flash of his bottom front teeth, during which my dentist detected tartar—the brittle substance that forms when plaque (a layer of bacteria) hardens, eventually causing tooth decay.

My heart sank, but he told me, "It is unlikely to have led to damage at this stage. I sometimes give children a scale and polish to get rid of it, but because this is his first visit it would be too overwhelming for him."

We arranged another appointment for six months' time in the hope Felix would be more compliant then.

If his junior patients need extensive dental work, my dentist sends them to specialist children's dentist (also in private practice) who is experienced in performing fillings on children as young as two. I asked this doctor how I can make brushing my children's teeth less traumatic. "Use star charts, bribery and begging, all the strategies to get a child to do something they don't want to," he advised. "Try and make it fun—let your children choose their toothbrush. Let them use an electric tooth brush if they want. Stand behind them with your hand under their face and give them a cuddle as you clean their teeth. Allow them to start brushing if they want to, before you carry on." While child-friendly toothpastes like strawberry are also available, my kids like them even less than the standard mint.

The evening after our visit to the dentist, chastened by the plaque developing on my son's teeth, I was determined to embark on an adequate cleaning session. Rosie, enthused by the princess-decorated toothbrush my dentist had given her, managed to endure a full two minutes. Felix, alas, ran away before I resorted yet again to the headlock technique. But he insisted on taking his new pirate toothbrush to bed and his last words before falling asleep were "I go to the dentist again soon." I live in hope.[12]

Finding a Pediatric Dentist (cont'd)

Most people find their own dentist. It's usually somebody who is close by, and convenient, or referred by a family member or a friend. If you are happy and comfortable with this dentist, ask him/her if they would feel comfortable seeing your child, and if not (this is not a failing on their part, but is the sign of a respectable and honest dentist) if he knows some other dentist who can treat your child.

Many people today look on the internet to find an appropriate doctor. But you must be wary. Numerous offices proclaim they love and treat kids, and they give the impression that they are children specialists when in fact even though they treat many kids, they do not have the proper training. In such cases, ask if the dentist is a certified specialist. But the best way to find a pediatric dentist in Canada is through The Canadian Academy of Pediatric Dentistry (CAPD), which is the membership organization representing over 300 pediatric dentists across Canada. Their members serve as primary and comprehensive oral health providers for thousands of children from infancy through adolescence. With specialized techniques of behaviour management and dental care they provide the diagnostic, preventive, therapeutic and consultative expertise required by children, including those with special care needs.

Whether you are looking for general information related to your child's oral health or guidance on a specific issue, you have come to the right place! The Membership Directory will allow you to find Pediatric Dentists in your city or town and you are urged to contact a specialists with your concerns: http://www.capd-acdp.org/Findakidsdentist

In each Province you can also call the provincial dental college for a listing of specialists.

In the U.S.A. it is best to call the AAPD website: http://www.aapd.org/

Note: if a dentist is not listed in CAPD/AAPD or the pertinent dental college, then they are not certified specialists.

You can also call local hospitals that treat kids with emergencies, call orthodontists who know dentists who routinely treat children.

Now, in many rural areas, there are no pediatric dentists to be found. To contact the one nearest you: call a local university that has a dental department—they will have dentists who treat children. Local hospitals that have dentists on staff will be able to treat your child or will refer you to qualified people. Other dental specialists in your area, orthodontists for example, deal with young people and will direct you to appropriate doctors.

Materials Used to Fill Children's Teeth

There are a multitude of different materials available. All have pros and cons: from silver to white plastic; to stainless steel crowns; to stainless steel crowns with white facings; or to white zirconium crowns.

Silver fillings are still used in filling back teeth and are more durable than white fillings. They are also applied in mouths that are more cavity-prone. And when the fillings to be placed are large, silver may be the material of choice. There is no definitive proof of any medical problems associated with this type of filling material.

White fillings are always used in the front teeth for cosmetic purposes, as the appearance of silver is unacceptable. White fillings are made of a tough plastic that needs to stand up to heavy forces. The advantage of white fillings is that they can be bonded to stick to the enamel, whereas silver fillings only hold by physical retention.

In the past, when cavities were large, the filling material of choice was stainless steel crowns. The material is well known for its durability, but there are now other choices available, in that you can get crowns with white plastic coating or crowns done in white zirconium. These are more expensive and you should be aware that large fillings on baby teeth tend to break down prematurely, and may need to be done over. Price is, therefore, a definite factor.

As mentioned, when repairing front teeth, fillings usually need to be done in white composite, for cosmetic purposes. However these teeth are small and take a lot of stress, and if the cavity is large a crown is the treatment of choice. You can ask for either a white crown or silver crown with white facing.

To do white fillings we need to have the child co-operate, as any salivary contamination during placement of the filling will lead to premature loss. A pediatric dentist will know what to do in this situation. Note: I do not recommend replacing silver fillings with white fillings if there is no breakdown of the filling. In other words the white filling should not be done strictly for cosmetic purposes.

More on Why to Treat Baby Teeth

Baby teeth are treated for various reasons: they play an important part in your child's appearance, teeth affect the sound of speech, they have an important part to play in growth and development of jaws, and they are used in chewing and mastication. Besides, untreated DC always deteriorates causing pain and suffering, and may end up with your child not eating properly. DC can also lead to infections that will harm permanent teeth and/or affect general health.

The best indicator that you are going to have a lot of dental caries, is caries at a young age. But not all teeth need fillings. Some just need to be monitored, especially if incipient. Others will need to be extracted, even if they are going to fall out in 6-12 months, because if left untreated, caries will go from decaying baby teeth, to decaying newly erupted permanent teeth. Only your pediatric dentist can assess the situation and come up with the best plan for your child.

Early treatment is usually not complicated. And it can keep your child from having to have baby teeth taken out prematurely. This is something you really want to avoid, because premature loss of baby teeth leads to growth and development problems, space loss and crooked permanent teeth. The crooked teeth are more difficult to clean, making them cavity prone and allowing the DC to attack secondary teeth.

Sometimes a child does not develop a permanent tooth and the baby tooth must serve as permanent. Pain in baby teeth is as painful as pain in permanent teeth, so it is truly important to take good care of the baby teeth your child has.

Many people think babies are too young for dental fillings, but delaying treatment leads to any DC deteriorating, and instead of dental fillings the teeth may end up requiring extractions, root canal treatments and crowns. But if the decay is minor, it can easily be treated by an experienced pediatric dentist in the office. Extensive work, however, will require the child to be put to sleep to have the work done. And, of course, more extensive work takes more time and, even with freezing, some pain and discomfort. The youngest child I have treated for dental caries was nine months of age.

Most parents are not aware that some baby teeth last until 12-14 years of age and leaving decayed baby teeth in the mouth when permanent teeth erupt will lead to early tooth decay on permanent teeth. And please remember that if a child is not compliant and will not or cannot cooperate for dental assessment, see a pediatric dentist. We are trained to deal with these situations.

And finally, if for no other reason, treat baby teeth early because the cost of neglect is expensive in both dollars and pain.

[12]http://www.telegraph.co.uk/women/mother-tongue/11785186/My-children-refuse-to-brush-their-teeth.html

Chapter 5
Initial Exam

There are several types of dental exams and valuations.

You may come in for an emergency visit because of a major concern or because your child is having pain in a certain area. The dentist will do an assessment of the specific situation or tooth that is likely to be the cause of the problem, and he or she may not necessarily evaluate any other treatment that might be necessary, although it is a given he/she will look around the whole mouth.

Or you may come in to see the dentist for a specific problem, in which case he will evaluate the cause and possible treatment of the problem. Typically no other assessment is done, although he/she may alert you to other possible concerns.

Then, there is the initial assessment that is a full assessment of the health and or disease in the oral cavity, which includes possible treatments and comments regarding any future treatment that may be necessary. This should involve a detailed medical and dental history, full intraoral and full-face exams, and the going over of any medical or mental or physical concerns. Necessary radiographs will be taken at this assessment to assist in full diagnosis. An initial exam is not just a caries count, but a full assessment of child's oral needs and it must be age specific.

You may have the same cavity on a tooth on a 3 year-old, 5 year-old, 9 year-old and a 12 year-old, and all may require different treatment according to the child's needs and development.

Many times a parent complains that the dentist didn't do anything, and is unhappy with the fees charged for a seemingly wasted appointment. However, the initial assessment is the most important part as assessing the right treatment is very important. A doctor with less experience and knowledge might recommend that the teeth are beyond repair and suggest extraction. However, the teeth may be saved, not only that, but premature extractions may lead to space loss and other developmental problems that do not show up for several years and can be very difficult and expensive to treat in the future.

The assessment and treatment plan are the most important part. Why is it important to have a good dental assessment? You may complain of your child's bleeding gums, and a hygienist may conclude that it is a gingivitis and may suggest that you need to brush the teeth better, but an experienced dentist would be aware of a differential diagnosis that can include bleeding disorders, other dental problems, viral infection or even possible leukemia. What you are paying for is all that expertise that you cannot see or evaluate. But I cannot stress this enough: you cannot do proper treatment unless you have a proper assessment from someone with both skill and knowledge.

There is a joke that explains this well ... *At a carnival a young lady sits down for a caricature drawing that takes 10 minutes, but the artist charges her $50 for the portrait. She was happy with the portrait but complains that she only sat in the chair for 10 minutes and was charged $50. The artist asked if she was happy, and when she told him she was, he explained that she was paying for the 5 years of training to be able to do such excellent portraits of such obvious quality.*

Thus, it is important as to who does the exam and evaluation, and the doctor's experience and knowledge is indeed important, because you want the best possible doctor for your kids.

The exam is important, but who does the exam and what is his/her expertise is even more important. After all, it is not about the fillings to be done, but ultimately what is the best treatment and long-term dental program for your child. It may be confusing for a parent, but you need to ask for explanations of what the doctor is going to do and why and what are the alternative treatments?

* * *

Recently I saw a child for a second assessment, as the parent was not happy with the dentist's treatment plan. This was a 3-year-old child, who he was going to put to sleep and do expensive crowns on all the upper front teeth. In addition to the cost of the dental treatment, the anesthetic fee to be included was to be just short of $5000. A quick assessment of the front teeth revealed that in fact no treatment at all was necessary. The teeth were not carious but worn down by the child grinding her teeth, there was no pain, and in fact if fillings had been placed, the child would have fractured them very quickly due to her grinding. So, what is that assessment worth—not only in money, but also in putting a child through a needless and difficult procedure that was most likely to fail? In this day and age, where all information is available to anybody on the Internet, it is important to evaluate the information, the evaluator being the critical factor

Other times I have seen cases where the dentist chose to leave teeth that were infected but not painful. He decided to not extract them in timely fashion and thus caused infection damage to the developing permanent teeth.

Frequently, the dentist will extract infected teeth and not place a spacer to hold space for the permanent successor. This results in the loss of space so that there is no place for the permanent successor to erupt. A situation like this requires braces to correct or possibly even extraction of the tooth as it can never find its proper place in the arch; being malposed it acts as a food trap and causes decay on adjoining teeth

The Value of a Proper Assessment is Invaluable

The assessment should not just be a caries count, there should also be an investigation as to why the child is getting dental caries and to determine what to do to stop the reoccurrence. This should be discussed even before treatment begins.

In the initial assessment, with age and development of the child being a factor in the treatment, things to be evaluated include the child's caries susceptibility level (which factors into the full treatment plan), the co-operation level of the child to withstand dental treatment and to follow the preventive program set out. Other things to be assessed are any pathology, from swellings, bumps, discolorations or other anomalies that may impact on the child's health.

Potential problems that do not yet exist but which can be prevented through proper care, such as a severe crowding problem that could lead to breakdown of these teeth due to difficult access with a toothbrush, could possibly be avoided with early assessment. Eruptive problems of baby and permanent teeth that come in too soon, or too late need to be assessed as to why and what are the implications.

In the caries assessment, the dentist must look for deep grooves on the molars, as they are more prone to decay than normal. The same goes for any crowding and rotation of teeth that make them difficult to clean.

What about the diet, soft drinks, sugary snacks, frequency of use and abuse? And for infants, is there any history of night feeding? Sometimes poorly developed enamel or "soft teeth" can be caught early before they decay and through early implementation of a proper preventive program the dental caries can be avoided. Any fevers or infections at a young age may disrupt normal tooth development, and medications given at a young age can affect developing teeth. For example, if you take tetracycline before the age of 13 it can and will cause permanent discoloration of any developing teeth, discoloration that cannot be corrected with whitening of teeth by normal means. Young adults and teen-age girls on birth control medication need to inform their dentist, as it may cause gum problems. Any information given to the dentist is confidential, and cannot be released even to the parent.

All sorts of other medications can cause problems in the mouth, so you need to tell your dentist all medications, even if you think it does not affect your dental treatment. For example a drug to control seizures, Dilantin causes severe swelling of the gums. And patients who are on long-term antibiotics can contract yeast infections in the mouth.

People with kidney problems may have problems with proper development of teeth as kidney problems affect the metabolism of calcium and phosphate that are needed in proper development.

A proper assessment takes into account missing teeth: Are they missing or are they late in eruption and development? And is this in the normal time frame, or is there another problem like the tooth is actually missing? Are there any extra teeth? Have 2 teeth tried to erupt into the same space, leaving a space because they have blocked each other from coming in? Timely and appropriate x-rays can confirm this. Interestingly both missing teeth and extra teeth are genetic in nature and may run in families.

The doctor may need to take dental x-rays to complete diagnosis, from finding dental caries between the teeth that are not visible or to determine if developing teeth are present and growing in properly. He/she may need to do a biopsy and caries assessment tests if indicated.

Although not mentioned and very rare, the dentist is also checking for any anomalies, like cancer, or precancerous conditions in the mouth, and he will do appropriate tests, or send the child to an appropriate clinic for further evaluation.

Another reason to go to a dentist who is familiar with working with kids is that I recently saw a teen-ager who had many missing teeth and who had extensive work done to replace her missing teeth, including braces to upright and straighten the existing teeth and implants to replace the missing teeth. As it was here in Ontario, Canada there is a government program that helps and pays for treatment of children with missing teeth, but the case must be assessed by the dentist, and sent to proper channels. Note at least 9 teeth need to be missing, thus somebody with 2-3 missing teeth is not eligible. If this teenager would have been seen by the right person, most of the treatment might have been covered.

Even at a young age, an orthodontic assessment should be carried out. Some treatments may need to be done at an early age or the situation may deteriorate and may need interceptive treatment or braces in the future. If this is the case, any early extraction of baby teeth can make a bad situation worse. Thus, even if you may need braces in the future, but your baby's teeth are not properly cared for and they are taken out prematurely, you may also need to have permanent teeth taken out as part of the orthodontic program.

Assessment for the need and timing of treating misaligned jaws and crooked teeth is important as well. Sometimes a timely interceptive orthodontic treatment can treat the problem, or proper timing of interceptive treatment can simplify a complex orthodontic case.

Children with Special Needs

Children with special needs usually have other more important concerns that require professional attention and that can take up a lot of parental energy. Whether the needs are physical or mental, these children can be challenging for a dental professional who does not have the training and experience to deal with the special management of the dental and preventive needs of these children.

In cases such as these, dental concerns are many times an afterthought, and as these kids may have communication issues, the problems may not come to the attention of the care giver until the situation is well deteriorated and requires extensive work, often under general anesthesia (when a timely visit to a dentist could have prevented these problems). These kids, especially, should be seen early by a pediatric dentist for a full oral assessment, to prevent unnecessary dental treatment, or to at least address issues before they can cause harm.

Offices will need special access for wheel chairs, not just ramps to get into the office, but the operatory must be wheel chair accessible to be able to treat these patients. Also it would be helpful if the dentist has a hospital affiliation, as any extensive work, especially with sedation and general anesthesia, should be carried out in a hospital or at least a hospital setting. This is to deal with possible post-operative concerns.

Children with special needs need routine care, just like everyone else, rather than waiting for a problem to show up. Remember, by the time you can see dental caries it may already be time for comprehensive treatment, as many more lesions may be present and only detectable on a thorough evaluation. Many of these kids have communication issues, and you may not be aware that the child is in pain. Look for change in eating or chewing patterns, drooling, resistance to letting you look or touch or brush in a certain area. It's also important to realize that such a child may have large dental caries and have no pain. So, this does not mean that treatment is not necessary.

Some of the older kids can be very violent and difficult to control in an office setting. These children may need to be seen at an institutional setting where they can safely be restrained and examined in a safe and healthy fashion.

Unless you go to an experienced pediatric dentist who routinely deals with special needs kids, they may get under treated or, conversely, over treated. The whole child needs to be evaluated, and not just the dental condition. Also, treatment needs to be carried out in a safe and timely fashion, taking the child's needs and medical risks into consideration. In many instances the dentist is unable to do a full and complete assessment, as the child will not co-operate to have dental x-rays, and even if they do get x-rays, they are often of a poor quality as the child may not be able to sit still long enough. However, if the child can sit in the chair, an attempt should be made. Many times the child can surprise you.

Emergency Exams

If the child is in pain or discomfort, an emergency exam is necessary, and you should contact your dentist. Sometimes it is difficult to assess pain in infants and young children, as just because a child is crying it does not necessarily mean they are in pain, or that the dental condition is causing pain.

There are also different types of pain, from chronic, long acting, acute, to very painful, spontaneous and stimulated pain.

Chronic pain may start with mild pain and discomfort and may last weeks and even months. This type of pain may get worse and progress to acute pain or it may go away if the cause is cleared up, or if the infection finds a way to drain and relieve pressure. Chronic pain in infants may be from teething, inflamed gums, infections and swellings. During teething, even if the child is not crying, he/she may start drooling, putting hands in the mouth and undergo a change in eating patterns.

In older kids, 6-12 years, it may be loose baby teeth ready to fall out, or it may be dental caries, or even food impacting between teeth, pushing on gums. There may also be pain on brushing, but you must be aware that some children do not like to get their teeth brushed and will cry and fuss when you attempt to brush teeth. I have seen children with soft teeth, that is where the enamel is not properly formed, and these teeth can be very sensitive to brush.

Teeth can be sensitive to hot and cold food or pain on eating and chewing hard foods. This may be due to dental caries, gum infection, viral infection, erupting teeth, or trauma due to a previous accident. The pain may persist, or go away, however the child should be assessed before the situation becomes acute in nature. Acute pain is uncontrollable, severe pain usually difficult to manage with painkillers. Any spontaneous pain that starts without provocation or starts at night needs attention as soon as possible. Also, any unusual swelling or discoloration of gums and teeth needs evaluation.

It is usually not a good idea to go to hospital emergency department for dental emergencies, because you will be seen by a doctor (who would normally be unfamiliar with dental problems), and even if they have a dentist on staff, you may wait hours until your child is seen. Instead, call your dentist. They will always give an emergency priority. In other words, do not wait until evenings and weekends to attend to your child's needs. The dentist will fit you in as soon as possible and will refer you to the hospital should the situation warrant such a visit.

Unfortunately, in young children, infections and swellings can deteriorate quickly—much faster than in an adult. In fact, if you wait until the next morning to see someone, you may need to go to the hospital in the middle of the night. Large swellings can be fatal if you get airway obstruction, and large swellings can cause fever. This means the infection is out of control and needs immediate attention. It should be noted, however, that dental infections rarely cause fevers, but if they do, immediate attention is necessary.

Sports injuries and other accidents should be seen as soon as possible to assess the injury—whether it is a broken tooth, or a fractured jaw. For example, if your child gets injured and gets a baby tooth knocked out, he or she needs to be seen by a dentist, as most doctors cannot tell a baby tooth from an adult tooth. If the tooth is knocked out, please try and find it. If it is a permanent tooth, time is of the essence, and the patient should be seen by a dentist ASAP! You see, if the tooth is a permanent tooth, the ideal thing to do is replace it into the socket that it was knocked out from. Placement does not need to be perfect, it can be crooked or even backwards but failing that, put the tooth between the gums and the cheek and bring the child to the dentist. Note: if the tooth has been out of the socket for more than one hour, prognosis is not good for long-term retention of the tooth.

A baby tooth should never be implanted again, however you need to bring your child to the dentist to see if there are any fragments left in the jaw. In young kids who fall, you may look and not find the tooth, because the tooth may have been pushed up into the jaw, an assessment, and necessary x-rays may be needed to ascertain if tooth was intruded. If the tooth cannot be accounted for, the child may need to be sent to hospital for a chest x-ray to see if child swallowed the tooth, or if it went down into the lungs.

Why Should You See a Pediatric Dentist (cont'd)?

The answer is special training. I teach at university and dental students have no, to very limited, experience with very young children and they do not have any training with treatment of infants. Family doctors have no experience and knowledge about diseases and infections or conditions in the mouth. On the other hand, Pediatric dentists go for specialized training after dental training for between two and three years. This training includes dealing with all issues that affect the mouth, studying the growth and development of jaws, learning diseases of infants and the special medical conditions that can adversely affect growth and development of the child.

Pediatric Dentists are set up to treat infants and their needs in case of trauma, infection, developmental problems, drug doses, prohibited drugs, infants with special needs and disabilities, setting up preventive programs that are age appropriate and may also have access to hospital in case hospital treatment is necessary.

One other thing to remember: not all orthodontists or oral surgeons will deal with dental issues of very young children, Pediatric Dentists will.

And finally ... Your children are your most valuable possession: do you want them treated by an inexperienced dentist who, for example, may do inappropriate procedures or psychologically harm your child by using inappropriate restraints? If your child suffers a traumatic experience, he/she will not forget it soon and will be much more difficult to handle for future dental treatment. Many adults have been scared by such negative dental experiences and never recover. How to pick the right dentist is the whole point of this book.

Chapter 6
Dental Treatment for Infants, Children and Teenagers

Although you may have the same cavity on the same tooth in children of different ages, treatment will probably be completely different, according to the age of the child, and the stage of tooth development. Remember, we treat children ... not teeth.

Dental Treatment One to Three Years

Most children at this age do not yet have dental caries, except for extenuating circumstances, like if they have soft teeth or they are night feeding. In fact, 90% of dental caries at this age is due to night feeding and 10% or less is due to soft teeth. And, as in the general population, we have the 80/20 rule, where 20% of the kids get 80% of the caries.

Incipient lesions or decalcifications (the start of dental caries) if caught early can be monitored and controlled so that the caries do not enlarge. The affected child should be seen regularly on a one to three month basis: to check for good oral hygiene; to instruct both parent and child about the necessary oral hygiene; to monitor the progress of the decay; and to determine if there is a need for a fluoride application. Of course, a lot will depend on co-operation of the child, and willingness of the parent to persist brushing under difficult circumstances. The idea is to prevent the caries from progressing quickly and perhaps even delay treatment if possible as, at this age, any extensive treatment will have to be done under general anesthesia.

Small caries can be treated in the office if the child is compliant, the caries are not too large or the affected teeth too numerous.

White fillings are bonded to the teeth, and it is imperative that the teeth stay dry all during the procedure, because if any contamination occurs, the filling will fail prematurely. Thus, if extensive work is to be carried out, the child will need to be sedated or put to sleep, to complete the work. Note: if the child is sedated or asleep, all the work is done at one sitting.

Also, a few words about sedation ... for young children it is ideal to use intravenous sedation, provided by a doctor or a dentist trained in IV sedation, with another dentist to do the actual fillings. Some dentists use oral sedation, which is completely different from IV sedation. Oral sedation is not as effective as IV sedation, as the child will be semi-conscious and still able to combat the dentist. Therefore, to protect the child, he or she will need to be restrained for their own safety, usually by a papoose board and wrap that restricts their movement. But the child is still fully awake, and feels the effects of treatment. I feel it is more dangerous to sedate a child deeply with oral sedation than IV, because it is easy to cross over the line from therapeutic effect to dangerous or fatal repercussions if there is an overdose, and it is more difficult to manage than an IV.

Dental Treatment Three to Seven Years

All of a child's 20 primary (baby) teeth usually break through the gums (erupt) between the ages of six months and three years. Then the permanent teeth begin to emerge, usually starting at about age six. Your child probably had his or her first trip to the dentist at twelve months of age, and now you probably have regular appointments set up. If for some reason your child has not yet seen a dentist, make an appointment for an exam.

- Your three to seven year-old child will be busily developing language skills and exploring the ever-widening world. Hard as it is to get a preschooler to sit still, this is the age during which you can teach good dental health habits.
- Your child can learn how to brush his or her own teeth at about three years of age and should be brushing his or her own teeth, morning and night, by age four, with parental help as needed. You should still supervise and check for proper cleaning.
- Give your child a small, soft toothbrush, and apply fluoridated toothpaste in an amount about the size of a small green pea. Encourage your child to watch you and older siblings brush teeth. A good teaching method is to have your child brush in the morning and you brush at night until your child masters the skill. Teach your child not to swallow the toothpaste.
- Start flossing your child's teeth as soon as they touch each other. You may find plastic flossing tools helpful. Talk with your dentist about the right timing and technique to floss your child's teeth and to teach your child to floss.
- If your four year-old sucks his or her fingers or thumb, help him or her to stop. If the child can't stop, see your dentist. A children's dentist (pediatric dentist) is specially trained to treat this problem. For more information, see the topic Thumb Sucking.
- Give your child nutritious foods to maintain healthy gums, develop strong teeth, and avoid tooth decay. These include whole grains, vegetables, and fruits. Try to avoid foods that are high in sugar and processed carbohydrates, such as pastries, pasta, and white bread.
- Discuss your child's fluoride needs with your dentist. If your child needs extra fluoride, your dentist may recommend a supplement or a gel or varnish that he or she would apply to your child's teeth. Use supplements only as directedand keep them out of reach of your child. Too much fluoride can

stain a child's teeth. It can even be toxic.
- Keep your child away from cigarette smoke (secondhand smoke). Tobacco smoke may contribute to the development of tooth decay and gum disease. As your child grows, teach him or her about the dangers of smoking and secondhand smoke.[13]

Dental Treatment Seven to Twelve Years

It is a well-known fact that dental caries is a significant health problem among people of all ages, but the magnitude of the problem is greatest among young children. A survey was carried out in 1590 children from 20 schools in both rural and urban areas in India. Out of this number 796 were male and 794 were female children. The overall prevalence of dental caries was 65.6%. High prevalence of dental

caries was seen in urban school children of seven to twelve years of age. The oral hygiene status was observed to be poor in rural school children, yet dental caries prevalence was higher in urban female children even with good oral hygiene. Also prevalence of dental caries was higher in urban school children even with good oral hygiene.

I would speculate that the lower evidence of dental caries in rural areas was due to lack of sugar in their diets. This is backed up by my own experience that children in this age bracket consume more sugar than their younger counterparts and thus experience more caries. Thus, regular check-ups and cleaning become very important.

Also, healthy dentition is a primary prerequisite for physical, social, emotional and psychological development and the well-being of a child. Early recognition of this disease is of vital importance to preserve oral health.[14]

Hospital General Anesthesia

The safest place to carry out deep sedation and general anesthesia is in a hospital, or hospital-like environment. Why - because things can go wrong and accidents and mishaps take place. If they do, the safest environment is in a hospital or hospital-like setting where they have all the medications and equipment to deal with emergencies.

The risk factors to be taken into account when thinking of putting a child to sleep are: the patency of the airway; severe asthma or other pulmonary or breathing problems; chubby children; kids who have special needs, medically or physically; a hereditary factor like Malignant Hyperthermia. All these kids can be treated safely without a problem in a hospital, or hospital-like setting, with the appropriate dentist, anesthesiologist, recovery room and recovery room staff.

Although there are risks for severe asthma procedures, they are extremely safe when carried out by a qualified doctor in an appropriate setting, and thousands are done routinely without any adverse effects.

Having Dental Work While Under General Anesthesia

When a child is put to sleep to have dental work completed all the caries need to be treated, even the small lesions. Be prepared to have even more dental caries diagnosed, as the dentist will probably take x-rays while the child is asleep and any cavities found will need to be treated.

While having a child/infant put to sleep for dental work is an extremely difficult procedure for the parents, it is more difficult for them than for the child. It is also a costly procedure with the extensive amount of dental work done and the anesthetic fees.

Many parents ask me to please only do the worst teeth, or fix only the front teeth. The problem with that is you cannot do a partial operation, if you do only the worst teeth, you will find that you will need to return soon to treat the small lesions that have now become large, because dental caries progress and deteriorate. Thus you will need to have a second procedure done to correct these teeth, and you will need to pay for another anesthetic fee, as well as go through the traumatic procedure again. With respect to filling the front teeth only, this is not advisable, because these teeth are lost relatively early (from five to eight years old) and the molars are not lost until 10-13 years. In addition, any premature loss of baby molars will lead to loss of space, and potential crowding when the permanent teeth erupt, which will make oral hygiene difficult, leading this area and these teeth to be cavity prone—or you can correct this crowding with braces at a hefty fee at a later date. Thus, repairing the back teeth is very important, and should be restored if at all possible.

Postoperative Care

Immediately, post-surgery kids wake up disorientate, and uncomfortable, as their mouths feel strange, and frozen, thus they cry but are not in any pain, and usually settle down quickly once the parent arrives. Postoperative stays in the hospital can be from 1-2 hours, depending on the length and complexity of the case. It is important to have all medications expelled, or have the effects fully gone. Kids can be given some soft food if they tolerate it.

What to expect: Most parents think the child will be in pain for days even weeks after surgery. The truth is that happens only if you get severely impacted wisdom teeth extracted. This can lead to long postoperative healing and discomfort for a week. With pediatric surgery and fillings this is not the case. The child will experience mild discomfort immediately, but will be able to eat comfortably the same day of the surgery and do any activities the next day, from going to school to sporting events. There may be some discomfort, but nothing that cannot be treated by a dose of Tylenol, or Advil. Most children return happily to the dental office for the post op evaluation. It should be stressed that brushing should be resumed the day after surgery. Many parents back off and do not want brush the teeth as they think it is painful. But this is not so; you should start brushing vigorously the next day and even if you find that the gums bleed, you must persist. The post op appointment will assess treatment, and stress the need for good oral hygiene.

Any child that has undergone dental treatment under general anesthesia, I usually see again in three months to assess oral hygiene and to check to see if the parents are keeping teeth clean. If not, we can still intercept the development of dental caries and before they have to develop a more intensive oral hygiene program. If you wait until six months have passed to return for assessment, my experience has been to find many kids with new caries that need to be repaired and sometimes enough decay for a second hospital intervention.

Repair versus Extracting Primary Teeth

If at all possible, the treatment of choice is always to repair at this age. The dentist should go over all options and go over pros and cons of each treatment. This should be done when you get the estimate and not the day of the surgery. Most teeth can be repaired by filling, however, badly broken down teeth will need to be repaired with crowns, if they are to last. The reason for this choice is that teeth that are badly broken down will not retain large fillings; crowns have a much higher success rate. Teeth should only be extracted as a last resort at this age. And this should happen only if the tooth is totally broken down and beyond repair or if the tooth is badly infected and possibly damaging the developing permanent tooth underneath. Crowns for the back teeth are made of stainless steel and are of a silver color. Crowns for the front teeth are also made of stainless steel, but these crowns are white.

[13]http://www.webmd.com/oral-health/tc/dental-care-3-years-to-6-years-topic-overview

[14]http://www.researchgate.net/publication/220000442_Oral_Hygiene_Status_of_7-12_year_old_School_Children_in_Rural_and_Urban_population_of_Nellore_District

Chapter 7
Other Needs

When to See an Orthodontist

You may have had discussions with your dentist regarding the benefit of having healthy teeth and proper jaw alignment. Crooked teeth are hard to clean and maintain. This can result in tooth decay, worsen gum disease and lead to tooth loss. Occlusion (bite) problems can contribute to abnormal wear of tooth surfaces, inefficient chewing function and excessive stress on the gum tissue and the bone that supports the teeth.

My feeling is that you should pursue an evaluation by an orthodontist whenever you have a concern or your dentist has a concern regarding you or your child's bite or jaw alignment. In fact, treatment by an orthodontist can be less costly than the additional care required to treat dental problems arising as a result of a malocclusion (improper bite).

When and Why to Straighten Teeth and Align Jaws

An orthodontist is a dentist with additional clinical training to treat malocclusions (improper bites), which may result from tooth irregularity and jaw issues. Both heredity and environmental factors can create crooked teeth and bite problems. Heredity factors include crowded teeth, teeth where there is too much space and malocclusions. Crooked teeth can be caused by thumb sucking and tongue thrusting as well as accidents occurring to the jaw.

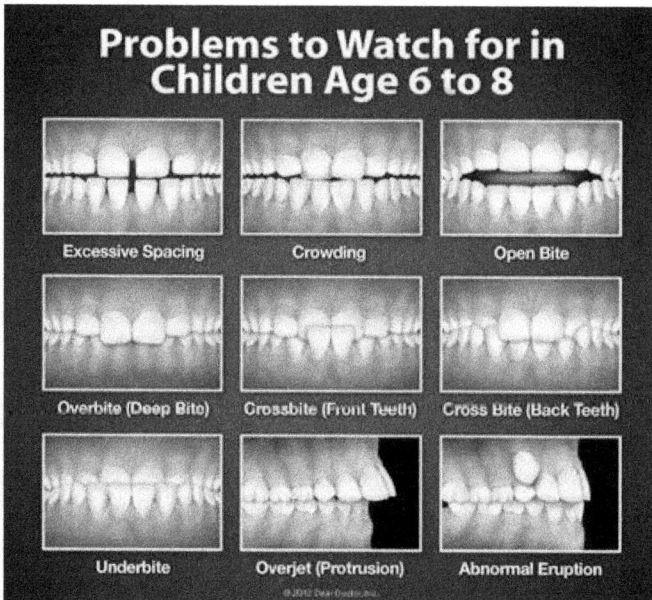

What are the Treatment Options to Straighten Teeth or Malocclusions?

There are three stages of orthodontic treatment. The first is when appliances are used to gain space in the mouth. For example, palatal expanders are used to expand the width of the palate and lingual bars are used to expand the lower jaw. The active corrective stage is next when the braces are placed on the teeth. The teeth are then adjusted and then straightened and malocclusions are corrected over a period of time based upon the severity of the teeth and jaw issues. The third stage is the retention stage after braces are removed and when the teeth are monitored through the use of a retainer (removable or fixed), and semi-annual orthodontic visits are conducted to maintain the straightened smile.

Braces

Tiny brackets are placed onto the front surface of the tooth and are made of metal or ceramic. The brackets are bonded to the front tooth surface with a glue-like material and metal bands can be used on the back teeth. Arch wires are placed inside the brackets and are made of a heat-activated nickel-titanium source that can become warm due to the temperature in the mouth, which will allow it to apply constant pressure on the teeth as well as when the arch wires are adjusted at the orthodontist's office.

Another newer alternative to braces is the Invisalign® system which uses a series of clear, removable aligners that are worn during the day and night to help in moving teeth into the correct alignment. When eating or brushing and flossing, the aligners may be removed.

Caring for Braces

Your orthodontist, dentist or dental hygienist will provide you with thorough instruction of how to properly clean your braces. Brushing should be conducted at least 2-3 times per day at a 45 degree angle in a back and forth motion. Be sure to remove plaque at the gum line to prevent gingivitis (inflammation of the gum tissue). Be sure to angle the toothbrush at the gum line and then gently brush around the brackets to remove plaque and food debris.

It is very important to clean in between your teeth with a floss threader and floss, a stimudent (tooth pick cleaner) or a proxabrush (interproximal cleaning brush) if there is space between the teeth. Oral irrigators may be recommended to remove food debris and irrigate the gum tissue to remove disease and odor-causing bacteria that may be there if you have gingivitis. An antibacterial toothpaste and over-the-counter antimicrobial mouth rinses could also be used with the oral irrigator or alone.

After the Braces Come Off

After your orthodontist has determined that your braces can be removed, it is very important that a retainer (a plastic appliance) be worn during the day or night as recommended by them. The retainer can be cleaned with warm water or toothpaste and a toothbrush after you wear it and placed in a plastic container when not in use.

See your dental professional for a twice a year professional cleaning and the orthodontist for regular maintenance appointments.[15]

Teeth Whitening

When choosing an over-the-counter tooth whitening product, always consult your dentist. They can tell you whether the product is safe and how often you should be using it. Alternatively, you can arrange to have the whitening process done by your dentist or a qualified dental assistant. This could help to avoid any pain, irritation or enamel breakdown that can arise from use of teeth whitening products.

Pregnancy and Adolescence

Many adolescent females become pregnant each year, yet there is no concise guide for their dental treatment. In my opinion, when treating a pregnant adolescent (or an adult), the primary goal is to maintain a safe environment for both the fetus and mother. Untreated dental disease can compromise the health of the mother and unborn child; therefore, dental treatment should not be withheld. In complicated pregnancies, the dentist should contact the patient's obstetrician prior to providing treatment or prescribing medication. With proper technique, dental radiographs do not place the fetus at risk and should be taken if they are of potential benefit. Preventive care should be delivered throughout the pregnancy, and elective routine care is best delivered during the second trimester.

Emergency Care

- For a knocked-out permanent or adult tooth, keep it moist at all times. If you can, try placing the tooth back in the socket without touching the root. If that's not possible, place it in between your cheek and gums. Then, get to your dentist's office right away.
- For a cracked tooth, immediately rinse the mouth with warm water to clean the area. Put cold compresses on the face to keep any swelling down.
- If you bite your tongue or lip, clean the area gently with water and apply a cold compress.
- For toothaches, rinse the mouth with warm water to clean it out. Gently use dental floss to remove any food caught between the teeth. Do not put aspirin on the aching tooth or gum tissues.
- For objects stuck in the mouth, try to gently remove with floss but do not try to remove it with sharp or pointed instruments.

When you have a dental emergency, it's important to visit your dentist or an emergency room as soon as possible.

Here are some simple precautions you can take to avoid accident and injury to the teeth:

- Wear a mouth guard when participating in sports or recreational activities.
- Avoid chewing ice, popcorn kernels and hard candy, all of which can crack a tooth.
- Never use your teeth to cut things. Use scissors.

Most dentists reserve time in their daily schedules for emergency patients. Call your dentist and provide as much detail as possible about your condition.

Guideline on Management of Acute Dental Trauma

Well-designed and timely follow-up procedures are essential to diagnose and manage complications.

After a **primary tooth** has been injured, the treatment strategy is dictated by the concern for the safety of the permanent dentition. If determined that the displaced primary tooth has encroached upon the developing permanent tooth, removal is indicated.

Fixed or removable appliances, while not always necessary, can be made in order to satisfy parental concerns for esthetics or to return a loss of oral or phonetic function.

It is important to caution parents that the primary tooth's displacement may result in any of several permanent tooth complications. The risk of trauma-induced developmental disturbances in the permanent successors is greater in children whose enamel calcification is incomplete.

The treatment strategy after injury to a permanent tooth is dictated by the concern for vitality of the periodontal ligament and pulp. Subsequent to the initial management of the dental injury, continued periodic monitoring is indicated to determine clinical and radiographic evidence of successful intervention.

Initiation of endodontic treatment is indicated in cases of spontaneous pain, abnormal response to pulp sensitivity tests, lack of continued root formation or breakdown of periradicular supportive tissue. To restore a fractured tooth's normal esthetics and function, reattachment of the crown fragment is an alternative that should be considered. To stabilize a tooth following traumatic injury, a splint may be necessary.

Instructions to patients having a splint placed include:
1. consume a soft diet;
2. avoid biting on splinted teeth;
3. maintain meticulous oral hygiene;
4. use chlorhexidine/antibiotics if prescribed; and
5. call immediately if splint breaks/loosens.

An incomplete fracture

Definition: incomplete fracture (crack) of the enamel without loss of tooth structure.
Diagnosis: normal gross anatomic and radiographic appearance; craze lines apparent, especially with transillumination.
Treatment objectives: to maintain structural integrity and pulp vitality. General prognosis: Complications are unusual.

Crown fracture–uncomplicated

Definition: an enamel fracture or an enamel-dentin fracture that does not involve the pulp. Diagnosis: clinical and/or radiographic findings reveal a loss of tooth structure confined to the enamel or to both the enamel and dentin.

Treatment objectives: to maintain pulp vitality and restore normal esthetics and function. Injured lips, tongue, and gingiva should be examined for tooth fragments. When looking for fragments in soft tissue lacerations, radiographs are recommended. For small fractures, rough margins and edges can be smoothed. For larger fractures, the lost tooth structure can be restored.

General prognosis: The prognosis of uncomplicated crown fractures depends primarily upon the concomitant injury to the periodontal ligament and secondarily upon the extent of dentin exposed. Optimal treatment results follow timely assessment and care.

Crown fracture–complicated

Definition: an enamel-dentin fracture with pulp exposure.
Diagnosis: clinical and radiographic findings reveal a loss of tooth structure with pulp exposure.
Treatment objectives: to maintain pulp vitality and restore normal esthetics and function. Injured lips, tongue, and gingiva should be examined for tooth fragments. When looking for fragments in soft tissue lacerations, radiographs are recommended.

- Primary teeth: Decisions often are based on life expectancy of the traumatized primary tooth and vitality of the pulpal tissue. Pulpal treatment alternatives are pulpotomy, pulpectomy, and extraction.
- Permanent teeth: Pulpal treatment alternatives are direct pulp capping, partial pulpotomy, full pulpotomy, and pulpectomy (start of root canal therapy). There is increasing evidence to suggest that utilizing conservative vital pulp therapies for mature teeth with closed apices is as

appropriate a management technique as when used for immature teeth with open apices.

General prognosis: The prognosis of crown fractures appears to depend primarily upon a concomitant injury to the periodontal ligament. The age of the pulp exposure, extent of dentin exposed, and stage of root development at the time of injury secondarily affect the tooth's prognosis. Optimal treatment results follow timely assessment and care.

Root fracture

Definition: a dentin and cementum fracture involving the pulp.

Diagnosis: Clinical findings reveal a mobile coronal fragment attached to the gingiva that may be displaced. Radiographic findings may reveal one or more radiolucent lines that separate the tooth fragments in horizontal fractures. Multiple radiographic exposures at different angulations may be required for diagnosis. A root fracture in a primary tooth may be obscured by a succedaneous tooth.

Treatment objectives: Primary teeth: Treatment alternatives include extraction of coronal fragment without insisting on removing apical fragment or observation. It is not recommended to reposition and stabilize the coronal fragment or if the tooth is not loose.

Concussion

Definition: injury to the tooth-supporting structures without abnormal loosening or displacement of the tooth. Diagnosis: Because the periodontal ligament absorbs the injury and is inflamed, clinical findings reveal a tooth tender to pressure and percussion without mobility, displacement, or sulcular bleeding. Radiographic abnormalities are not expected.

Treatment objectives: to optimize healing of the periodontal ligament and maintain pulp vitality.

General prognosis: For primary teeth, unless associated infection exists, no pulpal therapy is indicated. Although there is a minimal risk for pulp necrosis, mature permanent teeth with closed apices may undergo pulpal necrosis due to associated injuries to the blood vessels at the apex and, therefore, must be followed carefully.

Subluxation

Definition: injury to tooth-supporting structures with abnormal loosening but without tooth displacement.
Diagnosis: Because the periodontal ligament attempts to absorb the injury, clinical findings reveal a mobile tooth without displacement that may or may not have sulcular bleeding. Radiographic abnormalities are not expected.
Treatment objectives: to optimize healing of the periodontal ligament and neurovascular supply.
• Primary teeth: The tooth should be followed for pathology.
• Permanent teeth: Stabilize the tooth and relieve any occlusal interferences. For comfort, a flexible splint can be used. Splint for no more than two weeks.
General prognosis: Prognosis is usually favorable. The primary tooth should return to normal within two weeks. Mature permanent teeth with closed apices may undergo pulpal necrosis due to associated injuries to the blood vessels at the apex and, therefore, must be followed carefully.

Lateral luxation

Definition: displacement of the tooth in a direction other than axially. The periodontal ligament is torn and contusion or fracture of the supporting alveolar bone occurs.
Diagnosis: Clinical findings reveal that a tooth is displaced laterally with the crown usually in a palatal or lingual direction

and may be locked firmly into this new position. The tooth usually is not mobile or tender to touch. Radiographic findings reveal an increase in periodontal ligament space and displacement of apex toward or though the labial bone plate.

Treatment objectives:

- Primary teeth: to allow passive or spontaneous repositioning if there is no occlusal interference. When there is occlusal interference, the tooth can be gently repositioned or slightly reduced if the interference is minor. When the injury is severe or the tooth is nearing exfoliation, extraction is the treatment of choice.
- Permanent teeth: to reposition as soon as possible and then to stabilize the tooth in its anatomically correct position to optimize healing of the periodontal ligament and neurovascular supply while maintaining esthetic and functional integrity. Repositioning of the tooth is done with digital pressure and little force. A displaced tooth may need to be extruded to free itself from the apical lock in the cortical bone plate. Splinting an additional two to four weeks may be needed with breakdown of marginal bone.

General prognosis: Primary teeth requiring repositioning have an increased risk of developing pulp necrosis compared to teeth that are left to spontaneously reposition. In mature permanent teeth with closed apices, pulp necrosis and pulp canal obliteration are common healing complications while progressive root resorption is less likely to occur.

Intrusion

Definition: apical displacement of tooth into the alveolar bone. The tooth is driven into the socket, compressing the periodontal ligament and commonly causes a crushing fracture of the alveolar socket. Diagnosis: Clinical findings reveal that the tooth appears to be shortened or, in severe cases, it may appear missing. The tooth's apex usually is displaced labially toward or through the labial bone plate in primary teeth and driven into the alveolar process in permanent teeth. The tooth is not mobile or tender to touch. Radiographic findings reveal that the tooth appears displaced apically and the periodontal ligament space is not continuous. Determination of the relationship of an intruded primary tooth with the follicle of the succedaneous tooth is mandatory. If the apex is displaced labially, the apical tip can be seen radiographically with the tooth appearing shorter than it's contralateral. If the apex is displaced palatally towards the permanent tooth germ, the apical tip cannot be seen radiographically and the tooth appears elongated. An extraoral lateral radiograph also can be used to detect displacement of the apex toward or though the labial bone plate. An intruded young permanent tooth may mimic an erupting tooth.

Treatment objectives:
- Primary teeth: to allow spontaneous re-eruption except when displaced into the developing successor. Extraction is indicated when the apex is displaced toward the permanent tooth germ.
- Permanent teeth: to reposition passively (allowing re-eruption to its preinjury position), actively (repositioning with traction), or surgically and then to stabilize the tooth with a splint for up to 4 weeks in its anatomically correct position to optimize healing of the periodontal ligament and neurovascular supply while maintaining esthetic and functional integrity. For immature teeth with more eruptive potential (root 1/2 to 2/3 formed), the objective is to allow for spontaneous eruption. In mature teeth, the goal is to reposition the tooth with orthodontic or surgical extrusion and initiate endodontic treatment within the first three weeks of the traumatic incidence. Note: Root canal will be necessary.

General prognosis: In primary teeth, 90% of intruded teeth will re-erupt spontaneously (either partially or completely) in two to six months. Even in cases of complete intrusion and displacement of primary teeth through the labial bone plate, a retrospective study showed the re-eruption and survival of most teeth for more than 36 months. Ankylosis may occur, however, if the periodontal ligament of the affected tooth was severely damaged, thereby delaying or altering the eruption of the permanent successor. In mature permanent teeth with closed apices, there is considerable risk for pulp necrosis, pulp canal obliteration, and progressive root resorption. Immature permanent teeth that are allowed to reposition spontaneously demonstrate the lowest risk for healing complications. Extent of intrusion (seven mm or greater) and adjacent intruded teeth have a negative influence on healing.

Extrusion

Definition: partial displacement of the tooth axially from the socket; partial avulsion. The periodontal ligament usually is torn.
Diagnosis: Clinical findings reveal that the tooth appears elongated and is mobile. Radiographic findings reveal an increased periodontal ligament space apically.
Treatment objectives:
- Primary teeth: to allow tooth to reposition spontaneously or reposition and allow for healing for minor extrusion.[16]

Dental Insurance

In Canada, general oral health care is not included in the Canada Health Act. Most Canadians receive dental care through privately operated dental clinics and pay for services through insurance or by paying for it themselves.

According to the latest oral health component of the Canadian Health Measures Survey (CHMS):

- 62% of Canadians have private dental insurance;
- 78% of respondents from the higher income bracket have private insurance coverage
- 53% of adults between 60 and 79 of age do not have any dental insurance.
- 50% of respondents from the lower income bracket do not have any dental insurance.
- 6% of Canadians have public insurance. Some dental services are covered through government dental programs.

Dental insurance plans vary as much as do general medical insurance and drug care programs. It is quite common to see plans that provide for at least one regular visit to your dentist and that cover basic care like cleanings, fillings and extractions. Most plans only offer partial coverage of major dental care like crowns, root canals, dental plates and braces.

ACA (Affordable Care Act)

The **Patient Protection and Affordable Care Act (PPACA),** commonly called the **Affordable Care Act (ACA)** or colloquially **Obamacare**, is a United States federal statute signed into law by President Barack Obama on March 23, 2010. Together with the Health Care and Education Reconciliation Act amendment, it represents the most significant regulatory overhaul of the U.S. healthcare system since the passage of Medicare and Medicaid in 1965.

The ACA was enacted to increase the quality and affordability of health insurance, lower the uninsured rate by expanding public and private insurance coverage, and reduce the costs of healthcare for individuals and the government. It introduced mechanisms like mandates, subsidies, and insurance exchanges. The law requires insurance companies to cover all applicants within new minimum standards and offer the same rates regardless of pre-existing conditions or sex. In 2011 the Congressional Budget Office projected that the ACA would lower both future deficits and Medicare spending.

On June 28, 2012, the United States Supreme Court upheld the constitutionality of the ACA's individual mandate as an exercise of Congress's taxing power in the case *National Federation of Independent Business v. Sebelius.* However, the Court held that states cannot be forced to participate in the ACA's Medicaid expansion under penalty of losing their current Medicaid funding. Since the ruling, the law and its implementation have continued to face challenges in Congress and federal courts, and from some state governments, conservative advocacy groups, labor unions, and small business organizations. On June 25, 2015, in the case *King v. Burwell*, the Supreme Court affirmed that the law's federal subsidies to help individuals pay for health insurance are available in all states, not just in those which have set up state exchanges.

In March 2015, the Centers for Disease Control and Prevention reported that the average number of uninsured during the period from January to September 2014 was 11.4 million fewer than the average in 2010.[10] In April 2015, Gallup reported that the percentage of adults who were uninsured dropped from 18% in the third quarter of 2013 to 11.4% in the second quarter of 2015. [17]

According to the ADA (Americans with Disabilities Act)

• About three million children are expected to gain some form of dental benefits by 2018 as a result of ACA. Roughly one-third will gain Medicaid dental coverage and two-thirds will gain private dental coverage through health insurance exchanges and employer-sponsored plans. Combined, this will reduce the number of children who lack dental benefits by approximately 55 percent.

- Nearly 18 million adults will gain some level of dental benefits from the Affordable Care Act, but only 4.5 million of these adults are expected to gain extensive dental benefits through Medicaid. An additional 800,000 are expected to gain private dental benefits through health insurance exchanges. Combined, about 5 percent fewer adults will be without dental benefits. These increases will put pressure on the Medicaid system by generating an additional 10.4 million dental visits each year through Medicaid by 2018.
- Accountable care organizations could help bridge the gap between oral and general health care, improve coordination of dental care and help reduce overall health care costs. Dental care is not generally included as a core component within today's ACOs, but this is largely due to the current focus on Medicare populations.
- There is strong evidence that reforming Medicaid and increasing reimbursement rates to market levels would increase access to dental care. The Affordable Care Act does not do enough to address or solve administrative inefficiencies or low dental provider reimbursement levels seen at the state level.

[15]http://www.colgateprofessional.com/patient-education/articles/bringing-teeth-into-alignment

[16]http://www.aapd.org/media/Policies_Guidelines/G_trauma.pdf

[17] https://en.wikipedia.org/wiki/Patient_Protection_and_Affordable_Care_Act

Chapter 8
Final Summary

Beginning with the importance of primary teeth, Dr. Jack Maltz takes the reader on a journey, showing an up close and personal why you should be using a pediatric dentist for the children in the family. And he makes a convincing case.

Stressing that baby teeth affect the development of both the jaw and the adult teeth, Maltz demonstrates that dental caries (tooth decay) can and does happen to infants, giving a time table as to when to see the pediatric dentist and offering you simple instructions for cleaning the baby teeth.

Next Maltz shows you how dental caries starts, why and when to fix baby teeth and even describes a common risk factor approach for oral health. The importance of age-specific prevention is discussed along with specific steps that can be taken to avoid tooth decay. What happens when prevention doesn't work and how your insurance coverage fits into the situation are the final points in the chapter.

Dr. Maltz stops for a moment to answer the question WHY A PEDIATRIC DENTIST? This section also includes how to find a pediatric dentist in your area.

The core of this book deals with the initial exam, the differences in exams for variously aged children and, of course, exams for special needs and medically compromised children. These descriptions are followed by an overview of dental treatment for all ages of children, as well as specific issues like anaethesia and root canals.

Once the reader understands the reasoning behind various types of treatment, you are introduced to all the other needs, from emergency care to teeth whitening to aligning jaws. It's a fairly long list.

The whole point of the exercise was to show you, the reader, that your child can be best served by a pediatric dentist, but I have a surprise for you: The biggest reason for coming to a pediatric dentist is that we treat your most valuable family members. In fact, we treat children not teeth!

drjdentistry5@gmail.com

www.ingramcontent.com/pod-product-compliance
Lightning Source LLC
Chambersburg PA
CBHW062034200326
41519CB00017B/5037